Ophthalmology Revision Aid

To our wives

Ophthalmology Revision Aid

P T Khaw PhD MRCP FRCS FRCOphth DO
Consultant Ophthalmic Surgeon
Moorfields Eye Hospital and Institute of Ophthalmology, London

D S Hughes FRCS FRCOphth DO
Consultant Ophthalmic Surgeon
Hinchingbrooke and Addenbrooke's Hospitals, Cambridge

S J Keightley BSc FRCS FRCOphth DO
Consultant Ophthalmic Surgeon
North Hampshire Hospital, Basingstoke

R F Walters BSc FRCS FRCOphth DO
Consultant Ophthalmic Surgeon
University Hospital, Cardiff

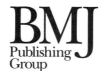
BMJ
Publishing
Group

© BMJ Publishing Group 1996

First published in 1996
by the BMJ Publishing Group, BMA House, Tavistock Square,
London WC1H 9JR

British Library Cataloguing in Publication Data

A catalogue record for this book is available from the British Library

ISBN 0–7279–1011–6

Typeset by Apek Typesetters Ltd, Nailsea, Bristol
Printed and bound in Great Britain by Latimer Trend Ltd, Plymouth

Contents

Acknowledgments

We would like to thank our many colleagues over the years who have helped us with their advice and criticism. In particular we would like to thank Professor Andrew Elkington for his encouraging support of the original book and we would also like to thank Vivian Balakrishnan (ocular motility), David Broadway (conjunctiva), David Charteris (retinal detachment and vitreous disorders), Francesca Cordeiro (medical ophthalmology and pharmacology), Jonathan Dowler (retinal vascular disorders, macula and Appendix I), Alex Foss (ocular tumours), Helena Frank (optics), David Gartry (cornea and sclera, and lens), Paula Gormley (uveitis and endophthalmitis), Tim Matthews (neuro-ophthalmology), and John Pitts (eyelids, orbit, and lacrimal system) for comments in their area of expertise. We would also like to thank Vicki King for her tremendous work and skill with the current manuscript and Peggy Khaw and Anna Quick for their help with the original book. Sarah Lawrence and the librarians at the Institute of Ophthalmology have been very helpful in getting references. Finally, we express our appreciation to Peter Jack who drew the diagrams.

Preface

This book is intended primarily as a revision text for those sitting examinations in ophthalmology. We have tried to strike a balance between basic science and clinical ophthalmology. It is also our hope that advanced medical students, optometrists, and ophthalmic nurses will find this book useful.

Our aim has been to provide a basic, pocket-sized text to which readers can add to create a permanent personal aide-memoire. By its very nature, it cannot be considered to be fully comprehensive but it may help readers to identify gaps in their knowledge and stimulate further reading. If any of the readers feel that we have omitted any important areas, please write to us and let us know.

PTK, DSH, SJK, and RFW
October 1995

1
EYELIDS

EYELID MARGINS

1 Palpebral aperture: 30 mm long $\times$ 10 mm high
2 Eyelid margins: divided into lateral $\frac{5}{6}$ and medial $\frac{1}{6}$ by lacrimal puncta:
  (a) lateral margin: 2 mm thick, rounded anterior edge, perpendicular posterior edge; grey line at junction of anterior and posterior lamellae—vascular watershed, splits easily with minimal bleeding
     (i) anteriorly: lashes—2–3 rows, longer in upper lid and in children, curved away from opposite lid, no erector muscles, 10 week growth, 5 month resting phase; glands of Moll—modified sweat glands, 2 mm long; glands of Zeiss—sebaceous glands, 2 per lash
     (ii) posteriorly: meibomian gland openings—25 upper lid, 20 lower lid
  (b) medial margin: both edges rounded, no lashes or glands; forms boundaries of lacus lacrimalis

ANTERIOR LAMELLA OF LID

1 Skin: fine texture, thin, and elastic; attached to deep fascia at medial and lateral canthus and at orbital margins; no subcutaneous fat
2 Orbicularis muscle:
  (a) three portions:
     (i) orbital: origin—medial palpebral ligament and adjacent bone; sweeps round lateral canthus
     (ii) palpebral: origin—medial palpebral ligament; sweeps across upper and lower tarsal plates (pre-tarsal) and orbital septum (preseptal); interdigitates to form lateral palpebral raphe
     (iii) lacrimal (Horner's muscle): origin—posterior lacrimal crest; fibres pass along the canaliculi to the tarsal plates extending to the lateral palpebral raphe
  (b) nerve supply: upper branches of VII entering deeply
  (c) function:
     (i) orbital—forcible closure of lids
     (ii) palpebral—blinking
     (iii) lacrimal—tear drainage

POSTERIOR LAMELLA OF LID

1 Tarsal plate: fibrous, scaphoid shaped skeleton of lid in which meibomian glands are embedded; 26 mm long × 10 mm (upper); 26 mm long × 4 mm (lower); stretches between palpebral ligaments and continuous with orbital septum; meibomian glands—10–15 acini around central duct producing oily secretion
2 Tarsal conjunctiva: tightly adherent to tarsal plate

ORBITAL SEPTUM

1 Extension of periosteum from orbital rim to tarsal plates
2 Preaponeurotic fat lies between it and the upper (levator palpebrae superioris) and lower lid retractors
3 Weaker inferiorly and superomedially (most common sites for herniation)
4 Pierced by levator palpebrae superioris, lower lid retractor, nerves, and vessels, e.g. frontal and supratrochlear nerves
5 Fuses with levator palpebrae superioris aponeurosis and lower lid retractor aponeurosis

LEVATOR PALPEBRAE SUPERIORIS

1 Origin: lesser wing of sphenoid
2 Insertion:
   (a) skin of lid (skin crease)
   (b) medial and lateral palpebral ligament
   (c) anterior surface of tarsal plate
   (d) pre-tarsal orbicularis
3 Relations:
   (a) lies above superior rectus
   (b) separated from orbital roof by IV and frontal division of trigeminal nerve
   (c) about 40 mm long ending 10 mm behind orbital septum in an aponeurosis
   (d) condensation running from trochlea to lacrimal gland (Whitnall's ligament)
   (e) fuses with septum 4 mm above tarsus
4 Function:
   (a) raises upper lid (about 12–17 mm in adults)
   (b) acts synergistically with superior rectus
5 Nerve supply—nerve III (upper division) entering deep surface.

MÜLLER'S MUSCLE

1 Origin: aponeurosis of levator palpebrae superioris
2 Insertion: upper edge of tarsus
3 Function: raises and "fine tunes" upper lid position (about ±2 mm)
4 Nerve supply: sympathetic via superior cervical ganglion

INFERIOR RETRACTOR

1 Forward extension of fascia from inferior rectus
2 Surrounds inferior oblique as Lockwood's ligament
3 Inserts into:
   (a) lower fornix
   (b) lower edge of tarsus
   (c) anterior surface of tarsus
4 Has smooth muscle component which lowers lower lid 1 mm

PALPEBRAL LIGAMENTS

1 Medial: 4 mm long and 2 mm wide; divides into anterior and posterior limbs that enclose the lacrimal sac; Horner's muscle runs with the posterior limb; anterior limb palpable, overlying inferior portion of lacrimal sac; angular vein lies superficially
2 Lateral: 7 mm long and 2 mm wide; separated from lateral palpebral raphe by palpebral portion of lacrimal gland

BLOOD SUPPLY TO EYELIDS

1 Arterial:
   (a) marginal arcade 3–4 mm from lid margin
   (b) deep peripheral arcade (upper lid only in some cases)
   (c) arcades formed from the medial and lateral palpebral arteries; anastomosis between intracranial and extracranial drainage
2 Venous: watershed and connection between intracranial and extra-cranial drainage

LYMPHATIC DRAINAGE OF EYELIDS

1 Submandibular nodes: drain medial $\frac{1}{3}$ of upper lid; medial $\frac{2}{3}$ of lower lid
2 Preauricular nodes: drain lateral $\frac{2}{3}$ of upper lid; lateral $\frac{1}{3}$ of lower lid

SENSORY NERVE SUPPLY TO EYELIDS

1 Upper lid: ophthalmic division of V (infratrochlear, supratrochlear, supraorbital, and lacrimal nerves)
2 Lower lid: maxillary division of V (infraorbital nerve)

FUNCTION OF LIDS

1 Protection of eye
2 Reconstitution of tear film
3 Coverage of eye during sleep

EXAMINATION OF EYELIDS

1 Lid height (palpebral aperture, scleral show, margin reflex distance)
2 Lid movement (levator function, lower lid retraction)

3 Muscle tone/lid attachments (orbicularis function, lid laxity)
4 Blinking and reflex movement (lagophthalmos, Bell's phenomenon, corneal sensation)
5 Contour and position (notching, ectropion, entropion)
6 Lid margin environment (blepharitis)
7 Tear film and function

BLINKING

1 Reflex:
   (a) sensory stimuli: latency 100 ms; persists in decerebrate state
   (b) optical stimuli: slower reflex due to central connections; absent in children; two aspects:
       (i) dazzle (subcortical)
       (ii) menace (cortical)
2 Voluntary
3 Spontaneous:
   (a) involuntary
   (b) rate: 12/min set by globus pallidus; reduced by alcohol; increased by emotion
   (c) amplitude 9·5 mm
   (d) duration 330 ms
   (e) total occlusion time 150 ms

EMBRYOLOGY

1 Eyelid folds form at 8 weeks of gestation
2 Upper lid formed by fusion of medial and lateral frontonasal processes
3 Lower lid formed by fusion of lateral maxillary processes and medial nasal processes
4 Lid folds meet and fuse at 12 weeks separating from nasal side at 24 weeks; plica forms at same time

CONGENITAL ABNORMALITIES

1 Ankyloblepharon: adhesion between lids (seen in pre-term neonates <26/40)
2 Ablepharon: absence of lids
3 Coloboma: notching of upper lid; associated with epidermoid cysts
4 Distichiasis: extra row of lashes from meibomian orifices directed backwards; treatment—lid split and posterior lamellar cryotherapy, trans-tarsal lash excision
5 Epicanthus: medial skin fold obscuring caruncle; most common congenital variation, especially in Mongoloid races; common cause of pseudoesotropia
6 Ptosis: 50% of all ptosis:
   (a) simple: unilateral; dystrophy of levator palpebrae superioris with or without reduced superior rectus function; features:
       (i) absent skin crease

4

    (ii) frontalis overaction
    (iii) chin up head position
    (iv) amblyopia if ptosis causes occlusion; surgery after 4 years if uncomplicated
  (b) double levator palsy: unilateral; features:
    (i) ptosis
    (ii) hypotropia
    (iii) failure of upgaze
    (surgery includes vertical transposition of the horizontal recti ±inferior rectus recession and ptosis correction)
  (c) jaw winking: unilateral ptosis; paradoxical elevation on jaw movement due to synkinesis with pterygoid muscles; surgery if marked (levator transection and brow suspension)
  (d) blepharophimosis: autosomal dominant; bilateral ptosis with inverted epicanthus, ectropion, and wide intercanthal distance
  (e) palsy of nerve III, aberrant regeneration, and Horner's syndrome
7 Ectropion: rare
8 Entropion:
  (a) bilateral, mild, affecting lower lid
  (b) especially in Mongoloid races
  (c) hypertrophy of skin and orbicularis
  (d) self limiting by 2 years
  (e) treatment: excision of strip of skin and orbicularis if lash/cornea contact marked

ACQUIRED DISORDERS

Entropion

1 Involutional:
  (a) affects lower lid
  (b) pathology:
    (i) preseptal overriding pre-tarsal orbicularis
    (ii) horizontal lid laxity due to stretched canthal tendons, orbital fat atrophy
    (iii) weakened tarsus allowing flexure
    (iv) vertical instability due to dehiscence of retractors
  (c) treatment:
    (i) taping of lid eversion sutures or botulinum toxin injection if unfit for surgery
    (ii) surgical correction of any or all above features, e.g. the Weis or Jones operations:
      • lid shortening in area of maximum laxity
      • lid split to evert and create scar preventing orbicularis overriding
      • lower lid retractor tightening
2 Cicatricial:
  (a) affects upper or lower lid
  (b) pathology: scarring and shortening of posterior lamella

(c) causes:
   (i) trachoma
   (ii) Stevens–Johnson syndrome
   (iii) radiation
   (iv) chemical injury
   (v) topical medications
   (vi) surgery
   (vii) trauma
   (viii) mucous membrane pemphigoid
(d) treatment of upper lid entropion
   (i) minimal: anterior lamellar reposition with or without lash removal
   (ii) moderate: as for minimal + tarsal groove
   (iii) severe: tarsal split, 180° rotation, or posterior lamellar graft
(e) treatment of lower lid entropion:
   (i) the Jones type procedure
   (ii) posterior lamellar mucous membrane or hard palate graft
3 Acute spastic:
(a) pathology: spasm of orbicularis with ocular irritation or essential blepharospasm; associated with involutional entropion
(b) treatment:
   (i) removal of irritation
   (ii) treatment of associated involutional entropion
   (iii) injection of botulinum toxin into orbicularis
   (iv) partial nerve VII section

Ectropion

1 Involutional:
(a) usually lower lid
(b) pathology:
   (i) horizontal lid laxity (canthal tendon and/or tarsal plate stretching)
   (ii) orbicularis weakness
(c) treatment:
   (i) cicatrisation by cautery
   (ii) conjunctivoplasty
   (iii) horizontal lid shortening, e.g. wedge resection or tarsal strip procedure
2 Cicatricial:
(a) upper or lower lid
(b) causes:
   (i) trauma: lacerations, burns, surgery
   (ii) tumours
   (iii) infections
   (iv) topical medications
(c) treatment:
   (i) prevention of exposure
   (ii) release of scarring, e.g. Z-plasty, skin grafting

3 Paralytic:
   (a) lower lid ± lagophthalmos
   (b) causes: myopathy or nerve VII disorders
   (c) treatment:
        (i)   prevention of exposure and corneal drying, e.g. botulinum induced ptosis
        (ii) tarsorrhaphy, medial canthoplasty, lid shortening procedures
        (iii) circlage, lid weights, and magnets
        (iv) nerve transposition or graft
        (v)   temporal muscle transfer

Ptosis

1 Neurogenic:
   (a) nerve III palsy
   (b) Horner's syndrome
   (c) jaw winking
   (d) aberrant nerve III regeneration
2 Myogenic:
   (a) congenital
   (b) acquired:
        (i)   myasthenia gravis—variable fatiguable ptosis; Cogan's twitch sign on upgaze
        (ii) myotonic dystrophy—autosomal dominant; bilateral ptosis
        (iii) mitochondrial myopathy—bilateral ptosis with ophthalmoplegia
3 Aponeurotic:
   (a) dehiscence of levator aponeurosis
   (b) causes:
        (i)   degenerative/senile
        (ii) trauma
4 Mechanical:
   (a) tumours
   (b) inflammations, e.g. vernal catarrh, blepharochalasis syndrome

Assessment of ptosis
1 History: onset, progression, variability
2 Exclude pseudoptosis, e.g. microphthalmos, cornea plana, or hypertropia in eye with "ptosis" or lid retraction, prominent eye, hypotropia in other eye
3 Measure levator function (immobilise frontalis): normal: > 12–17 mm
4 Measure degree of ptosis: palpebral aperture and margin reflex distance
5 Check ocular motility and pupil function
6 Ask patient to move jaw (jaw winking)
7 Check Bell's phenomenon, corneal sensation, tear film, and tear secretion
8 General examination: consider Tensilon test

Treatment of ptosis
1 Treat underlying condition, e.g. anticholinesterases in myasthenia gravis

7

2 Surgery: proportional to levator function and degree of ptosis
3 Tear substitutes with myogenic causes of ptosis as higher risk of corneal exposure
4 Spectacle props (ptosis crutches), haptic contact lenses

Infections and inflammations of the eyelids

1 Stye (external hordeolum): infected gland of Zeis
2 Chalazion (internal hordeolum): chronic inflammation of a meibomian gland associated with blepharitis:
  (a) histopathology: lipogranuloma with foreign body giant cells, fibrosis, and fluid content
  (b) treatment:
    (i) conservative—hot compresses and topical antibiotics
    (ii) surgery—incision and curettage
3 Blepharitis:
  (a) inflammation of the lid margin
  (b) types:
    (i) infection/infestation (staphylococci, *Demodex folliculorum*)
    (ii) seborrhoeic (diphtheroids, *Pityrosporum ovale*)
    (iii) rosacea associated
  (c) symptoms: ocular irritation
  (d) signs:
    (i) erythema and telangiectasis of lid margin
    (ii) meibomianitis—passive retention of inspissated secretions, chalazia, and styes
    (iii) trichiasis, madarosis, poliosis
    (iv) tear film instability and debris; greasy scales at lash roots (seborrhoea); collarette type scales (staphylococcal)
    (v) corneal pannus, punctate epithelial erosions, marginal keratitis, phlyctenulosis
  (e) treatment:
    (i) lid hygiene/massage
    (ii) lubricants
    (iii) topical antibiotics ± steroid
    (iv) systemic antibiotics, e.g. oxytetracycline
4 Occasional infections:
  (a) impetigo
  (b) erysipelas
  (c) pyogenic granuloma—granulation tissue related to bacterial infection
  (d) tuberculosis
  (e) syphilis
  (f) anthrax
5 Viral infections:
  (a) herpes simplex (primary and secondary)
  (b) herpes zoster
  (c) viral warts: filiform lesions; histopathology: parakeratosis, vacuolated nuclei with eosinophilic inclusions

    (d) molluscum contagiosum:
       (i) "water warts"—umbilicated contagious lesions associated with a follicular conjunctivitis
      (ii) histopathology: distended epithelial cells containing eosinophilic bodies which stain with Lugol's iodine
     (iii) treatment: expression and chemical cautery or excision
6 Fungal infections and infestations:
    (a) tinea infections (ringworm)
    (b) lice (pediculosis)
    (c) fly maggots (myiasis)
    (d) onchocerca nodules

Trichiasis

Backwardly directed lashes causing irritation; related to scarring of the eyelids.
1 Causes:
    (a) staphylococcal blepharitis
    (b) past herpes zoster ophthalmicus
    (c) trauma (physical, chemical, and irradiation)
    (d) conjunctival scarring diseases
2 Treatment:
    (a) epilation or soft contact lens
    (b) cryotherapy—double freeze–thaw to −20°C for large segments
    (c) electrolysis (hyfrecation) or argon laser for single lashes
    (d) local excision
    (e) surgery

Lagophthalmos (inadequate eyelid closure)

1 Associations:
    (a) race (Mongoloid)
    (b) nocturnal
    (c) nerve VII palsy
    (d) proptosis
    (e) lid retraction or scarring
    (f) buphthalmos
    (g) coma, e.g. severe dehydration
2 Treatment:
    (a) lubricants
    (b) lid taping, botulinum ptosis
    (c) surgery, e.g. retractor recession, tarsorrhaphy

Causes of reduced blinking

1 Drugs, e.g. alcohol
2 Reduced conscious level
3 Hyperthyroidism
4 Parkinson's disease
5 Progressive supranuclear palsy

Blepharoclonus

1 Exaggerated reflex blinking with increased frequency and contraction
2 Associations:
 (a) ocular irritation
 (b) tic

Orbicularis myokymia

1 Involuntary contraction resulting in an annoying twitching sensation
2 Related to fatigue and occasionally hemifacial spasm and multiple sclerosis

Blepharospasm

1 Involuntary tonic, spasmodic, bilateral eyelid closure; 60+ years; women > men
2 Causes:
 (a) idiopathic
 (b) Parkinson's disease
 (c) psychogenic
 (d) post-encephalitic
 (e) tetany
 (f) drugs, e.g major tranquillisers
3 Treatment: botulinum toxin injections into orbicularis oculi

Floppy lid syndrome

Unilateral or bilateral generalised laxity of lid tissues.
1 Symptoms: ocular irritation, redness
2 Signs:
 (a) superficial keratitis
 (b) easy distraction of lid from globe, easy upper lid eversion
 (c) ectropion of lower lid
 (d) ptosis and lash ptosis
3 Treatment:
 (a) wedge excision
 (b) canthal tendon repair

Causes of lid swelling

1 Local causes, e.g. allergy, infection
2 Blepharochalasis syndrome
3 Dysthyroid states
4 Nephrotic syndrome
5 Angioneurotic oedema
6 Premenstrual syndrome
7 Infiltrates, e.g. myeloma
8 Norrie's disease

Xanthelasma

Fatty plaques at medial end of the eyelids (usually bilateral).
1 Associations:
   (a) primary hyperlipidaemic states
   (b) diabetes mellitus
   (c) hypothyroidism
   (d) primary biliary cirrhosis
   (e) necrobiotic xanthogranuloma
2 Histopathology: foam cells (macrophages) in epidermis
3 Management:
   (a) exclude underlying cause
   (b) excision (60% recurrence)
   (c) laser ablation or chemical cautery

Benign tumours

1 Basal cell papilloma (seborrhoeic keratosis):
   (a) common, sessile
   (b) histopathology: basal cell proliferation with keratin nests
2 Squamous cell papilloma:
   (a) common, sessile, or pedunculated tumour
   (b) histopathology: excessive convoluted epithelium; central fibrovascular core; keratin horn formation
3 Solar keratosis:
   (a) flat, multiple, scaly lesions, occasionally papillomatous with horn formation; premalignant.
   (b) histopathology: dysplastic epithelium with pronounced keratosis, but no invasion
4 Keratoacanthoma:
   (a) enlarges over months, then regresses; volcano shaped with keratin plug
   (b) histopathology: difficult to differentiate from squamous cell carcinoma unless whole lesion examined histologically; hyperplastic epithelium; parakeratosis, hyperkeratosis; no invasion but basal inflammation
5 Haemangioma:
   (a) strawberry naevus: evident in neonatal period; grows then usually regresses by 5 years of age; may be either cutaneous, orbital, or mixed types
   (b) histopathology: proliferation of capillaries, some of which are not canalised
6 Neurofibroma:
   (a) associated with neurofibromatosis
   (b) histopathology: nodular proliferation of Schwann cells and fibroblasts; staining for S100 protein shows neuroectodermal origin
7 Naevi:
   (a) congenital collections of naevus cells; pigmented or non-pigmented; may develop pigmentation after puberty
   (b) histopathology: naevus cells stain uniformly blue with haematoxylin and eosin (H & E); classified according to location within skin:

11

   (i) epidermal—slightly thickened epithelium with naevus cells forming cysts

  (ii) junctional—activity at epidermal/dermal junction, occurring in children or at puberty

 (iii) dermal—fascicles of naevus cells within the dermis; diffuse dermal naevus or naevus of Ota associated with choroidal melanomas

 (iv) compound—malignant

Malignant tumours

1 Basal cell carcinoma:
- (a) most common malignant carcinoma
- (b) lower lid most common site
- (c) do not metastasise but invade locally
- (d) types:
  - (i) noduloulcerative: well defined; histopathology—palisaded basal cell proliferation with invasion and cyst formation; ulceration and inflammation
  - (ii) sclerosing (morphoea); histopathology—islands of basal cells infiltrating beneath epidermis; multifocal
- (e) treatment: depends on position of tumour and histological site, patient health, and preference:
  - (i) cryotherapy—10% recurrence rate; required modality in basal cell naevoid syndrome
  - (ii) radiotherapy—not for medial canthus, mid-upper lid and fornices or central lid
  - (iii) surgical—recurrence in only 25% of those with histologically incomplete excision; aim for 4 mm clearance or use Mohs' mapping technique

2 Squamous cell carcinoma:
- (a) arise *de novo* from premalignant states such as solar keratoses, arsenical keratoses, and xeroderma pigmentosum
- (b) may metastasise to lymph nodes
- (c) histopathology: depends on degree of differentiation ranging from well differentiated keratinising carcinomas (with cell nests and keratin pearls) to anaplastic spindle cell growths; may evoke a chronic inflammatory response
- (d) treatment: radical resection

3 Carcinoma *in situ* (Bowen's disease):
- (a) 5% of eyelid tumours
- (b) upper lid most common site; everted edges
- (c) histopathology: dedifferentiation of epithelial cells; changes are localised to epidermis; transition to squamous cell carcinoma may occur

4 Meibomian gland carcinoma:
- (a) rare
- (b) localised; may present as recurrent chalazion
- (c) diffuse: may present as persistent chronic blepharitis
- (d) histopathology: foamy vacuolated cells with hyperchromatic nuclei

(e) treatment: radical excision and radiotherapy
5 Carcinoma of gland of Moll:
  (a) very rare
  (b) extramammary Paget's disease
6 Malignant melanoma:
  (a) very rare
  (b) arising *de novo* or as a result of junctional change in a naevus
  (c) signs:
    (i) itching
    (ii) bleeding
    (iii) pigmentary changes
    (iv) change in size of an existing naevus
  (d) types:
    (i) lentigo maligna—superficial premalignant condition of elderly people
    (ii) superficial spreading
    (iii) nodular—occurs only in covered areas, not on face
  (e) prognosis: depends on site, depth of invasion (poor if invasion >1·5 mm) and degree of inflammation

Miscellaneous conditions

1 Cyst of Moll:
  (a) retention cyst
  (b) clear and fluid filled
2 Cyst of Zeis:
  (a) retention cyst
  (b) white cheesy material

13

2
ORBIT

ANATOMY

1 Pyramidal, volume about 30 ml
2 Height about 34 mm, width about 39 mm, depth about 45 mm
3 Constricted anteriorly; maximum diameter 1 cm behind rim (equator of globe in this position)
4 Anterior opening roughly square
5 Medial walls parallel; lateral walls perpendicular to each other
6 Medial and lateral walls intersect at 45°
7 Orbital axis 22·5° to the sagittal plane

Walls

1 Roof:
    (a) thin: made up of frontal bone, lesser wing of sphenoid
    (b) relations:
        (i) superiorly—frontal sinus, anterior cranial fossa
        (ii) anterolaterally—lacrimal gland depression
        (iii) anteromedially—trochlear depression (4 mm behind rim); trochlear spine in 10% of skulls
        (iv) anteriorly—supraorbital notch ($\frac{1}{3}$ from medial end)
2 Medial:
    (a) very thin (0·2–0·4 mm); made up of frontal, maxillary, lacrimal, ethmoid, and body of sphenoid bones
    (b) relations:
        (i) medially—nasal sinuses and anterior ethmoidal artery and nerve
        (ii) anteriorly—lacrimal fossa (anterior and posterior crests)
        (iii) superiorly—frontoethmoid suture (obliterated with age)
        (iv) posteriorly—optic canal
3 Floor:
    (a) thin (0·5–1·00 mm); made up of maxillary, zygomatic, and palatine bones
    (b) relations:
        (i) inferiorly—maxillary sinus; infraorbital foramen 4 mm below rim, $\frac{1}{3}$ from medial end

(ii) medially—fossa of inferior oblique insertion (inferolateral to nasolacrimal duct)
4 Lateral:
 (a) strongest, no relations to sinuses; made up of zygomatic bone and greater wing of sphenoid bone
 (b) relations:
  (i) anterolaterally—temporal fossa
  (ii) posterolaterally—middle cranial fossa
  (iii) superiorly—frontozygomatic suture (common site for dermoids)
  (iv) laterally—zygomatic foramina (zygomaticofacial and zygomaticotemporal nerves)
 (c) lateral orbital Whitnall's tubercle, 11 mm below frontozygomatic suture; insertion of:
  (i) lateral palpebral ligament
  (ii) lateral rectus cheek ligament
  (iii) levator aponeurosis
  (iv) suspensory ligament of globe

Contents

1 Globe
2 Orbital fat (intraconal and extraconal)
3 External ocular muscles
4 Nerves (II, III, IV, Va, VI, and sympathetic nerves)
5 Vessels (branches of ophthalmic artery, and superior and inferior ophthalmic veins)
6 Lacrimal gland

Superior orbital fissure

1 About 2 cm long
2 Relations:
 (a) superiorly: lesser wing of sphenoid
 (b) inferiorly: greater wing of sphenoid
3 Connects orbit with middle cranial fossa
4 Transmits III, IV, Va nerves, superior ophthalmic vein, and recurrent meningeal artery
5 Laterally occluded by dura and periosteum

Inferior orbital fissure

1 About 2 cm long
2 Relations:
 (a) superiorly: greater wing of sphenoid bones
 (b) inferiorly: palatine/maxillary and zygomatic bones
3 Connects orbit with infratemporal and pterygopalatine fossae
4 Separated from superior orbital fissure by neck of sphenoid
5 Traversed by maxillary nerve
6 Transmits zygomatic nerve, sympathetic fibres, and venous anastomosis
7 Largely occluded by periosteum

Branches of the ophthalmic artery

1 Central retinal artery
2 Posterior ciliary arteries:
   (a) about 15 short arteries
   (b) about 2 long arteries
3 Lacrimal artery

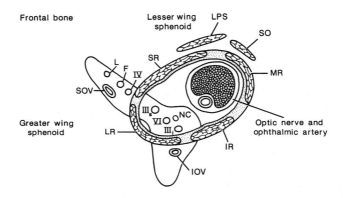

Figure 2.1 Superior orbital fissure (schematic diagram)
Key:
Above annulus of Zinn: SOV = superior orbital vein; L = lacrimal nerve; F = frontal nerve; IV = fourth nerve
Through annulus of Zinn: III_s = third nerve (superior division); NC = nasociliary nerve; III_i = third nerve (inferior division); VI = sixth nerve
Below annulus of Zinn: IOV = inferior orbital vein
Muscles: LPS = levator palpebrae superioris; SO = superior oblique; SR = superior rectus; MR = medial rectus; IR = inferior rectus; LR = lateral rectus

4 Recurrent meningeal branches
5 Muscular branches: anterior ciliary arteries
6 Supraorbital artery
7 Ethmoidal arteries:
   (a) posterior
   (b) anterior
8 Medial palpebral arteries:
   (a) superior
   (b) inferior
9 Terminal branches:
   (a) supratrochlear artery

(b) dorsal nasal arteries

Optic foramen

1 Transmits optic nerve and ophthalmic artery through sphenoid bone
2 Downward and outward at 36° to the midline
3 Lateral wall 5–7 mm
4 Roof 10–12 mm
5 Dura adherent to walls
6 Ophthalmic artery inferior then lateral to optic nerve
7 Medially: sphenoid sinus and posterior ethmoid air cells

Periosteum

1 Lines orbit
2 Adherent at sutures and foramina
3 Binds down superior oblique tendon
4 Thickened at orbital rim at insertion of orbital septum
5 Divides to enclose lacrimal sac
6 Continuous over superior orbital fissure and inferior orbital fissure

EMBRYOLOGY

1 Ethmoid, sphenoid: from cartilage
2 Frontal, lacrimal: from membrane
3 Maxilla, palatine, zygoma: from first branchial arch

ORBITAL SYMPTOMS

1 Globe position
2 Lid appearance
3 Diplopia
3 Visual impairment
4 Pain

ORBITAL SIGNS AND EXAMINATION

1 Proptosis: measure with exophthalmometer from lateral orbital rim to corneal apex; normal <20 mm; >2 mm difference between eyes significant; types:
  (a) axial: intraconal (dysthyroid eye disease most common)
  (b) non-axial: extraconal (95% tumours)
  (c) dynamic properties:
    (i) increase with Valsalva manoeuvre
    (ii) pulsation
    (iii) vascular lesion or defect in bony wall
2 Vision: may be impaired as a result of:
  (a) optic nerve compression caused by raised intraorbital pressure (tight septum) or direct pressure on, or infiltration of, the optic nerve; reduced colour vision an early sign

17

   (b) raised intraocular pressure
   (c) exposure keratopathy
   (d) choroidal folds
   (e) pseudohypermetropia
   (f) field defects
3 Strabismus:
   (a) ocular movements (±globe displacement, restrictive or paralytic palsy)
   (b) forced duction test (muscle tethering or contraction)
4 Palpation:
   (a) lumps and local swellings (check lacrimal gland)
   (b) tenderness
   (c) retropulsion of the globe
5 Reduced sensation in branches of Va and Vb
6 Auscultation: listen for bruit (e.g. caroticocavernous fistula)
7 Slitlamp:
   (a) tear film instability with exposure
   (b) superior limbic keratoconjunctivitis associated with dysthyroid eye disease
   (c) conjunctival vessels
      (i) arterialised (dural shunt)
      (ii) tortuous at muscle insertion (dysthyroid eye disease)
   (d) raised intraocular pressure particularly on upgaze
8 Ophthalmoscopy:
   (a) disc pallor
   (b) disc swelling
   (c) opticociliary shunts
   (d) choroidal folds
9 General examination

CAUSES OF PSEUDOPROPTOSIS

1 Ipsilateral:
   (a) high myopia
   (b) buphthalmos
   (c) orbital asymmetry
   (d) lid retraction
2 Contralateral:
   (a) enophthalmos
   (b) ptosis
   (c) microphthalmos

CAUSES OF PULSATILE PROPTOSIS

1 Caroticocavernous fistula
2 Large frontal mucocele
3 Meningoencephalocele
4 Arteriovenous malformation
5 Neurofibromatosis in children

RADIOLOGICAL VIEWS OF THE ORBIT

Superseded by ultrasound scans, computed tomography, and magnetic resonance imaging.
1 Caldwell's view: general view
2 Waters' view: orbital floor
3 Rhese's view: optic foramen
4 Lateral view/axial basal view: sinuses

PHLEBOGRAPHY

1 Not commonly used
2 Performed via frontal or angular vein
3 Outlines superior ophthalmic vein in 3 portions:
   (a) extraconal
   (b) intraconal above optic nerve
   (c) intraconal lateral to optic nerve
4 Apsidal veins connect with inferior ophthalmic vein
5 Inferior ophthalmic vein may not fill
6 Need to compare both sides

ULTRASONOGRAPHY

1 Produced by a piezoelectric crystal; the transducer transmits and receives 1000 times/s; frequency range: 5–20 MHz
2 Propagation through tissues depends on velocity, absorption, and frequency
3 Ultrasound is refracted, reflected, and absorbed by ocular and orbital structures
4 Reflected sound returning along the path of the propagated beam is recorded
5 A-scan: one dimensional; time–amplitude study
6 B-scan: two dimensional; sectional view with a scanning transducer
7 Ultrasonic probe coupled to ocular structures, using, for example, 5% methyl cellulose or by immersion coupling using waterbath
8 Ocular diagnostic applications:
   (a) posterior vitreous detachment
   (b) vitreous haemorrhage
   (c) retinal detachment
   (d) massive preretinal fibrovascular proliferation
   (e) intraocular tumours
   (f) intraocular foreign bodies
   (g) biometry
9 Orbital applications:
   (a) high reflectivity:
      (i) dysthyroid myopathy
      (ii) haemangioma
      (iii) neurofibroma
   (b) low reflectivity:
      (i) cyst

    (ii) mucocele
   (iii) varix
   (iv) lymphoma

COMPUTED TOMOGRAPHY

1 Investigation of choice in most orbital disease
2 Pixel size governs definition (volume averaging)
3 Slices either thick (3 mm) or thin (1·5 mm) and either contiguous or stepped
4 Axial slices normally parallel to Reid's baseline (external auditory meatus to inferior orbital rim)
5 Optic canal views best at angle of 30° to baseline
6 Coronal and sagittal views possible; reformatted image quality depends on slice thickness and separation
7 Contrast depends on tissue density; Hounsfield scale grades contrast (-1000 = air, 0 = water, $+1000$ = dense bone)
8 Intravenous contrast:
  (a) enhancement of normal vascular structures:
     (i) extraocular muscles
    (ii) lacrimal gland
   (iii) arteries and veins
   (iv) uveoscleral rim
  (b) essential extraorbital extension, e.g. intracranial
  (c) helpful with:
     (i) venous thrombosis
    (ii) cystic masses
   (iii) optic nerve tumours

MAGNETIC RESONANCE IMAGING

1 Investigation of choice in most intracranial disease
2 Intensity of signal dependent on hydrogen proton density, and T_1 and T_2 relaxation times
3 Surface coils increase resolution of orbital pathology
4 Advantages over CT scan:
  (a) no radiation
  (b) no elaborated patient positioning
  (c) less image degradation, e.g. dental fillings
  (d) good optic canal, chiasma, and differentiating optic nerve from adjacent masses; also differentiating flowing from clotted blood and inflammatory lesions.
5 Disadvantages compared with CT scan:
  (a) patient motion artefacts
  (b) poor spatial resolution
  (c) no signal from calcification
  (d) potential dangers with pacemakers and foreign bodies
  (e) higher cost

CONGENITAL ABNORMALITIES OF THE ORBIT

1 Early suture closure:
   (a) all synostoses: may produce hydrocephalus
   (b) oxycephaly:
       (i) all sutures closed
       (ii) tower skull
       (iii) proptosis (50%), visual failure, exotropia
   (c) brachycephaly: coronal suture closure
   (d) Crouzon's disease
       (i) brachycephaly and maxillary hypoplasia
       (ii) hypertelorism: shallow orbits, proptosis, exotropia, optic atrophy, irregular dentition, hooked nose
2 Primary or secondary underdevelopment of the orbit:
   (a) mandibulofacial dysostosis:
       (i) hypoplasia of mandible and zygoma
       (ii) shallow inferior orbital rim
       (iii) lower lid abnormalities, anti-Mongoloid slant
   (b) hypertelorism:
       (i) early ossification of sphenoid wings
       (ii) exotropia
   (c) hydrocephalus: shallow orbits, optic atrophy
   (d) micro-/anophthalmos: underdeveloped orbits
   (e) buphthalmos: large orbit

FACIAL FRACTURES OF THE ORBIT

1 Le Fort III: separation of face from cranium
2 Le Fort II: separation of central block of face from skull
3 Malar fractures: fractures involving zygomaticofrontal process, zygomatic arch, and maxilla; often displaced and requires open reduction

BLOW OUT FRACTURES OF THE ORBIT

1 Orbital floor/medial wall fractures resulting from blunt trauma; transmitted forces result in deformation and fracture
2 Pure; do not involve rim
3 Complicated; involve rim
4 Pure floor fracture may be linear or punched out with or without prolapse or incarceration of orbital contents
5 Clinical features:
   (a) suggestive history
   (b) enophthalmos, although may have proptosis
   (c) hyper- or hypoaesthesia of infraorbital area
   (d) surgical emphysema
   (e) limited ocular movements; may be due to:
       (i) oedema or haemorrhage within extraocular muscle
       (ii) nerve trauma
       (iii) entrapment of tissues
       (iv) hypoglobus or enophthalmos

    (f) rise in intraocular pressure on upgaze
    (g) nasal bleeding (unilateral)
6 Investigations:
    (a) assess ocular position (exo-/enophthalmos, hypoglobus)
    (b) field of binocular single vision, Hess (Lees) screen
    (c) CT scan (coronal sections):
        (i) fluid level in sinuses
        (ii) hanging drop sign
        (iii) look for fracture of orbital rim and medial wall
    (d) forced duction test
7 Management:
    (a) conservative
    (b) surgery: repair by 14 days after injury; extraocular muscle surgery should be delayed; indications for surgery include:
        (i) fracture involving the rim
        (ii) linear fracture and tissue entrapment
        (iii) enophthalmos >3 mm or hypoglobus
        (iv) diplopia in primary position
        (v) small field of binocular single vision
        (vi) positive forced duction test
    (c) principles:
        (i) repair defect with bone or non-autogenous material
        (ii) strabismus surgery may be required—inferior rectus recession (adjustable), or reverse Knapp procedure

OTHER ORBITAL FRACTURES

1 Orbital roof fractures: associated with sharp objects; danger of intracranial penetration and retained foreign bodies; blunt trauma to frontal area may result in linear fractures; these may involve the optic canal
2 Trochlear disinsertion:
    (a) sharp trauma
    (b) iatrogenic, e.g. while approaching ethmoidal artery in treatment of epistaxis

CAUSES OF ORBITAL HAEMORRHAGE

1 May be subperiosteal or intraorbital
2 Causes:
    (a) trauma: high risk of visual loss
    (b) spontaneous: varices, lymphangioma
    (c) iatrogenic: retrobulbar injection

CAROTICOCAVERNOUS FISTULA

1 Causes:
    (a) direct (communication between internal carotid artery and cavernous sinus)—usually trauma to sclerotic aneurysm (75%)

[handwritten margin note: diffuse enlargement of all EO muscles / CT — enlargement of SOV]

(b) dural (communication between dural branches and cavernous sinus)—usually spontaneous (25%)

2 Clinical features:
   (a) high flow:
      (i) pulsating exophthalmos
      (ii) bruit
      (iii) diplopia (limited eye movements) *↑ cav pressure*
      (iv) pain
      (v) conjunctival congestion and chemosis *(arterioligation of conj vessels)*
      (vi) increased intraocular pressure *(↑ episcleral venous pressure)*
      (vii) dilated conjunctival vessels, forehead veins, and choroidal vessels (arterialisation)
      (viii) visual impairment
      (ix) optic nerve ischaemia
      (x) intraocular hypoxia (rubeosis) *ocular ischemic syndrome*
   (b) low flow: as above but less severe
3 Prognosis: 5% spontaneous cure, 50% vision lost
4 Management:
   (a) conservative
   (b) neuroradiological balloon catheter embolisation *(interventional arteriography)*
   (c) internal carotid ligation

ACUTE ORBITAL INFECTIONS

1 Preseptal cellulitis:
   (a) lid oedema, erythema, and tenderness
   (b) orbital contents undisturbed
2 Orbital cellulitis:
   (a) features as above with reduced motility, proptosis, fever, and pain
   (b) aetiology:
      (i) spread from sinuses, dental abscess, or skin infection
      (ii) direct infection following trauma or surgery
      (iii) systemic infection
   (c) causes:
      (i) *Staphylococcus aureus* and *Streptococcus* spp. most common
      (ii) *Haemophilus influenzae* in children <3 years of age
   (d) complications:
      (i) central retinal artery or vein occlusion
      (ii) optic nerve inflammation
      (iii) cavernous sinus thrombosis
      (iv) brain abscess
   (e) management:
      (i) CT scan
      (ii) blood culture
      (iii) culture of any infectious site, e.g. conjunctiva, nasopharynx
      (iv) high dose intravenous antibiotics
      (v) nasal decongestants or sinus washout
      (vi) surgical drainage of abscess
3 Orbital abscess:
   (a) may be intraorbital or subperiosteal

    (b) associated with orbital cellulitis
4 Cavernous sinus thrombosis:
    (a) associated with orbital cellulitis
    (b) marked limitation of motility, visual loss, palsies of III, IV, V, VI
    (c) bilateral extension; oedema over mastoid (emissary vein)
    (d) fever, prostration
    (e) treatment: antibiotics, anticoagulants
    (f) prognosis poor

CHRONIC ORBITAL INFECTIONS

1 Causes:
    (a) tuberculosis
    (b) syphilis
    (c) fungal (*Aspergillus* and *Mucor* spp.)
2 Signs:
    (a) irreducible proptosis
    (b) orbital apex syndrome (ptosis, visual loss, internal and external ophthalmoplegia)

ORBITAL INFESTATIONS

1 Cysticercosis (larvae of *Taenia solium*)
2 Trichinosis (*Trichinella spiralis*)
3 Hydatid disease (*Echinococcus granulosus*)

DYSTHYROID EYE DISEASE

1 Associations:
    (a) hyper-/hypothyroidism although patient may be clinically euthyroid
    (b) thyroid acropachy, pretibial myxoedema (Graves' disease)
    (c) pernicious anaemia
    (d) myasthenia gravis
    (e) Addison's disease
    (f) HLA association varies with different populations
2 Aetiological theories:
    (a) uncertainty over exact aetiology
    (b) T cells active against common antigen (orbit and thyroid)
    (c) antibodies may activate T and B cells (thyroglobulin, thyroid microsomal, TSH receptor)
    (d) T and B cells may activate orbital fibroblasts resulting in self perpetuating inflammation
    (e) fibroblasts produce glycosaminoglycans that hydrate; fibrosis and tethering may result
3 Female:male ratio = 4:1; average age of onset 50 years; worse disease in smokers
4 Werner classification = NO SPECS:
    No symptoms or signs
    Only signs, e.g. lid retraction, lid lag, superior limbic keratoconjunctivitis

Soft tissue swelling, e.g. lid oedema
Proptosis:
(a) 21 mm taken as the upper limit of normal
(b) unilateral or bilateral
(c) septal tightness may play a role in preventing proptosis
Extraocular muscle involvement; most commonly inferior rectus and medial rectus; infiltrative and restrictive following fibrosis
Corneal ulceration
Sight loss:
(a) corneal ulceration
(b) optic neuropathy
(c) raised intraocular pressure
(apart from the first 2 grades all the others are subdivided into absent, minimal, moderate, and severe)
5 Histology:
(a) external ocular muscles: up to ×8 increased size as a result of lymphocytic infiltrate; later necrosis and fibrosis
(b) orbital fat: proliferation and mucopolysaccharide deposits
6 Investigations:
(a) thyroid function: T_3, T_4, TSH, and TRH test
(b) autoantibodies: including anti-thyroid microsomal, anti-thyroid stimulating globulin
(c) B-scan ultrasound
(d) CT scan: enlarged muscles and exclude other orbital pathology; tendon insertions are always spared
(e) biopsy: rarely required as diagnosis usually evident
7 Management:
(a) assess thyroid status; treatment of thyroid disorder may worsen ocular condition, e.g. radioiodine treatment
(b) corneal protection:
(i) lubricants
(ii) moist chamber
(iii) tarsorrhaphy (surgically or with botulinum toxin)
(c) intraocular pressure: reduce if raised
(d) systemic corticosteroids: for acute disease with optic nerve compression; immunosuppressive agents may be required
(e) radiotherapy (2000 cGy)
(f) orbital decompression (up to 3 wall)
(g) external ocular muscle surgery and/or injection of botulinum toxin into muscles
(h) lid retractor surgery ± blepharoplasty

PSEUDOTUMOUR

1 Definition: non-specific, non-neoplastic, polyclonal inflammation affecting any or all soft tissue components
2 Clinical features:
(a) middle aged women most commonly affected
(b) clinical picture depends on predominant site of involvement:

      (i) anterior
     (ii) lacrimal
   (iii) posterior
   (iv) diffuse
    (v) myositis
   (vi) orbital apex syndrome
  (vii) Tolosa–Hunt syndrome
(viii) bilateral—30% are children

3 Histology: polyclonal cellular infiltration with variable amount of fibrosis and no evidence of vasculitis
4 Management:
  (a) make histological diagnosis to exclude:
    (i) lymphoma
   (ii) polyarteritis nodosa, Wegener's granulomatosis, sarcoidosis, and Waldenström's macroglobulinaemia
  (b) systemic corticosteroids
  (c) radiotherapy

ORBITAL TUMOURS

1 Primary: 70%
2 Direct spread: 23%
3 Distant spread: 4%
4 Systemic disease: 3%

VASCULAR TUMOURS

Most common primary benign tumours.
1 Capillary haemangioma:
  (a) present in infancy
  (b) may be superficial (strawberry naevus), deep, or mixed
  (c) dynamic proptosis
  (d) initially increase in size; regress by 5 years
  (e) may cause astigmatism, amblyopia, or disfigurement
  (f) treatment by local injection of steroid or surgery
2 Cavernous haemangioma:
  (a) adults
  (b) slowly progressive, unilateral proptosis
  (c) intraconal with dilated cavernous; blood filled spaces within a capsule
  (d) treatment: surgical, excision
3 Lymphangioma:
  (a) rare; of unknown origin
  (b) fluid filled cystic spaces; may involve conjunctiva, eyelids, orbit, and oropharynx
  (c) slow growing infiltrative lesions; may increase in size with upper respiratory tract infections; may haemorrhage (chocolate cysts) and present acutely
  (d) treatment: large surgical debulking or drainage of chocolate cyst

4 Varix:
  (a) most common vascular abnormality
  (b) non-pulsatile proptosis, which may have increase on a Valsalva manoeuvre
  (c) phlebolith on CT scan
5 Haemangiopericytoma: very rare

NEURAL TUMOURS

1 Optic nerve glioma (juvenile pilocytic astrocytoma):
  (a) 4–8 years of age; 55% have neurofibromatosis
  (b) slowly progressive proptosis
  (c) fusiform optic nerve enlargement (intradural growth)
  (d) benign indolent hamartoma with astrocytic replacement of optic nerve
  (e) management usually conservative; surgical resection if tumour extends into optic canal; radiotherapy useful if tumour intracranial
2 Meningioma:
  (a) women > men, 40–50 years of age
  (b) primary or from intracranial spread, e.g. sphenoid ridge
  (c) slow growing, locally invasive
  (d) early visual loss before onset of proptosis
  (e) fundal signs:
      (i) optic disc swelling
      (ii) optic atrophy
      (iii) opticociliary shunts
  (f) histology: arises in arachnoidal tissue; syncytial arrangement of cells with psammoma bodies
  (g) Management is conservative or radical excision
3 Neurofibroma:
  (a) associated with neurofibromatosis
  (b) proliferation of Schwann cells, endoneural fibroblasts, and axons within nerve sheath
  (c) management: conservative or surgical debulking

LYMPHOMA

1 Age group: patients usually over 60 years of age
2 Types: range from benign lymphoid hyperplasia (polyclonal) to lymphoma (monoclonal)
3 Usually isolated in the orbit but exclude systemic disease, e.g.:
  (a) systemic lymphoma
  (b) leukaemic deposits
  (c) plasmacytoma
  (d) myeloma
4 Management:
  (a) biopsy for histological classification
  (b) staging:
      (i) general examination

(ii) blood count and peripheral blood cell markers

(iii) chest radiograph, whole body CT scan

(iv) bone marrow aspiration

(v) lymphangiography

(c) radiotherapy (10–30 Gy) usually adequate for isolated disease; chemotherapy if systemic

5 Prognosis: excellent for local disease

MESENCHYMAL TUMOURS

1 Benign: rare; of any orbital component; occasional sarcomatous change

2 Sarcoma associated with Paget's disease (1%) and orbital radiotherapy for retinoblastoma

3 Rhabdomyosarcoma:

  (a) clinical features

     (i) most common primary malignant tumour of children; arises in embryonal mesenchymal rests with potential to differentiate into striated muscle

     (ii) average age 7 years

     (iii) rapid growth of mass in superonasal quadrant

     (iv) non-axial proptosis

     (v) may have inflammatory appearance

  (b) types:

     (i) embryonal—most common in orbit

     (ii) alveolar

     (iii) pleomorphic—rare in orbit

     (iv) botyroid

     (v) differentiated

  (c) management:

     (i) biopsy to confirm diagnosis

     (ii) radiotherapy and chemotherapy

  (d) prognosis: 90% five year survival if respond

LACRIMAL TUMOURS

1 Fifty per cent are inflammations and lymphoid proliferations

2 Pleomorphic adenoma (benign mixed cell tumour):

  (a) tumour of epithelial origin

  (b) 20–60 years

  (c) painless, usually with long history (> 1 year)

  (d) palpable hard nodular mass

  (e) non-axial proptosis; reduced ocular movements; astigmatism

  (f) local pressure changes on CT scan (moulding)

  (g) histology: components of epithelial, myoepithelial, and connective tissue; irregular tubular formation with double layer epithelium; myxoid stroma; pseudocapsule

  (h) management: biopsy contraindicated; *en bloc* resection

  (i) prognosis: good if removed without rupturing the pseudocapsule

3 Carcinoma:
  (a) malignant tumours of epithelial origin
  (b) painful, usually short history (< 1 year)
  (c) ± sensory loss over distribution of lacrimal nerve
  (d) local bony erosion on radiograph
  (e) types: adenoid cystic, adenocarcinoma, and mucoepidermoid
  (f) management:
      (i) exclude infection with a 2 week course of antibiotics
      (ii) biopsy if no improvement
      (iii) radical local resection and radiotherapy
  (g) prognosis poor

LOCAL SPREAD FROM ADJACENT STRUCTURES

1 Nasal sinus carcinomas:
  (a) maxillary most common
  (b) non-axial proptosis, epiphora, epistaxis, infraorbital anaesthesia
2 Neglected skin tumours:
  (a) basal cell carcinoma
  (b) squamous cell carcinoma
3 Extraocular spread:
  (a) melanoma
  (b) retinoblastoma
4 Intracranial meningioma
5 Nasopharyngeal carcinoma

METASTATIC TUMOUR

Any systemic carcinoma can metastasise to the orbit. Proptosis, pain, and bony destruction common to all.
1 Neuroblastoma:
  (a) childhood
  (b) 40% develop orbital metastases
  (c) acute proptosis and lid ecchymosis
  (d) urinary vanillylmandelic acid raised
2 Acute leukaemia: may be the present with deposit in orbit (chloroma)
3 Breast: most common metastasis in women; scirrhous carcinoma may develop enophthalmos
4 Bronchogenic carcinoma: most common metastasis in men
5 Order of frequency (site of spread):
  (a) breast (orbital fat)
  (b) lung
  (c) prostate (bone)
  (d) melanoma (extraocular muscle)
  (e) gut
  (f) kidney

CYSTIC LESIONS

1 Dermoids:
  (a) clinical features:

      (i) children
     (ii) common, painless, slow growing
    (iii) upper, outer quadrant most common
    (iv) dermal structures trapped along suture lines during development; may extend intracranially

  (b) complications:
      (i) erosion to anterior cranial fossa
     (ii) ulceration, infection, rupture, chronic sinus formation

  (c) management: excision in all cases as leakage occurs resulting in inflammation

2 Mucocele of nasal sinuses:
  (a) develops from chronic sinus infection with obstruction to draining ostium
  (b) frontal and ethmoid sinuses most commonly affected
  (c) may invade orbit leading to proptosis
  (d) management involves drainage and obliteration of the sinus

3 Lipoepidermoid:
  (a) benign mass usually laterally with subconjunctival component
  (b) may have cilia in conjunctival component
  (c) management: conservative or excision of anterior element with care not to damage lacrimal ductules

4 Cholesterol granuloma: post-traumatic; inflammatory reaction to denatured intradiploic haemorrhage

3
LACRIMAL SYSTEM

LACRIMAL GLANDS

1 Main gland:
   (a) orbital portion makes up $\frac{2}{3}$ of gland; meniscus shaped, situated at superolateral angle of orbit; fixed to periosteum; 10–12 ductules to upper outer fornix; 1–2 to lower fornix
   (b) palpebral portion lies along ductules, separated from orbital portion by levator palpebrae superioris aponeurosis
   (c) histology: tubuloracemose gland, divided into lobules by fibrous septa attached to periosteum; double layer acini consisting of myoepithelial and cylindrical eosinophilic secretory cells
   (d) blood supply: lacrimal artery (branch of ophthalmic artery)
   (e) nerve supply of the lacrimal gland:
      (i) parasympathetic: secretomotor; superior salivatory nucleus via nerve VII, greater (superficial) petrosal nerve, pterygopalatine ganglion (synapse), zygomatic nerve (Vb), and lacrimal nerve (Va)
      (ii) sympathetic: vasomotor; superior cervical ganglion via deep petrosal nerve, pterygopalatine ganglion (no synapse), and zygomatic nerve (Va)
2 Accessory glands:
   (a) glands of Krause: isolated lobules in upper (40) and lower (6) fornices
   (b) glands of Wolfring: lobules at proximal ends of tarsal plates (3 upper, 1 lower)

DRAINAGE SYSTEM

1 Puncta: elevated and retroverted; 6 mm from medial canthus; fibrous ring maintains patency; increased prominence with age
2 Canaliculi: 2 mm vertical; 8 mm parallel to lid margin; joins fellow forming common canaliculus; enters lacrimal sac obliquely as valve of Rosenmüller; lined by stratified squamous epithelium
3 Lacrimal sac: 6×12 mm; lying in lacrimal fossa, invested by periosteum; superficial portion of medial canthal ligament anteriorly; fundus of sac (5 mm) lies above and the common canaliculus directly behind

the medial canthal ligament; angular vein medially (8 mm from medial canthus); sac slopes laterally and downwards to constriction at start of nasolacrimal duct (valve of Krause); lined by 2 layers of epithelium—columnar and flattened

4 Nasolacrimal duct: 15 mm long; lying in bony canal formed by maxillary and lacrimal bones; surrounded by rich venous plexus; passes backwards, laterally, and downwards, opening under inferior concha at physiological valve of Hasner

EMBRYOLOGY

1 Lacrimal gland: ectodermal origin as invagination from conjunctiva forming gland; connective tissue from mesenchyme

2 Lacrimal drainage apparatus: formed from buried cord of ectodermal cells between frontonasal and maxillary processes at the 12 mm stage, later canalising from above; nasolacrimal duct opens soon after birth

3 Canaliculi: formed from cord of cells during the formation of the lids; canalise from the sac to the lid; open at month 7 of gestation

TEARS

1 Fornix tears: static pool until full blink provides mixing

2 Marginal tears: brisk flow in meniscus to puncta

3 Precorneal tears: 5–8 μm thick; stable for 15–40 seconds; ruptures as result of lipid migration to mucous layer, particularly in areas of film thinning, resulting in a hydrophobic surface; blink heals rupture

The precorneal tear film

1 Mucin layer (deep layer): glycoprotein layer produced by conjunctival goblet cells (holocrine glands), glands of Manz (perilimbal), and crypts of Henle (proximal end of tarsal plates); adsorbed on to microvilli of corneal epithelial cells converting this to a hydrophilic surface

2 Aqueous layer (middle layer):
   (a) composition varies with age and lacrimal gland disease: 98·2% water, 1·8% solids (proteins), pH 7·35; if acid or alkali produces irritation; glucose concentration low; hyperosmolarity may produce some corneal dehydration; continuous production throughout the day; basal secretion = 2 μl/min; mucin and aqueous phase mix to form a single stable layer with reducing concentration of mucin more superficially.
   (b) causes of reflex aqueous secretion (>100 μl/min):
      (i) irritation
      (ii) yawning, coughing, sneezing
      (iii) psychic excitation, developing at 4 months of age
      (iv) photic (bright light)
      (v) crocodile (aberrant innervation of gland)
   (c) functions of the aqueous layer:
      (i) oxygenation—provides oxygen to corneal epithelium
      (ii) protection—dilution; washing away debris; non-specific anti-

bacterial agents, e.g. lysozyme and lactoferrin; specific bacterial agents, e.g. secretory IgA, IgG
  (iii) optical—smooth anterior refracting surface
3 Oily layer (outer layer): thin layer of low melting point cholesterol esters and lecithin produced by meibomian glands; aids vertical stability of aqueous phase, reduces evaporation, and prevents lid margin overflow

TEAR DRAINAGE

1 Conjunctival sac volume $= 35 \mu l$
2 Overflow of margins at $100 \mu l$
3 Evaporation of 10–50% of tear production
4 Tear pump:
  (a) capillary action into canaliculi
  (b) contraction of Horner's muscle creates siphoning action within canaliculi and expands sac sucking tears in
  (c) sac empties under the effect of gravity

KERATOCONJUNCTIVITIS SICCA

1 Symptoms:
  (a) redness
  (b) burning sensation
  (c) gritty sensation
  (d) "stiff lids": difficulty with initial opening
  (e) secondary epiphora in some cases
2 Signs:
  (a) meniscus size decreased
  (b) tear film debris: tear film break up time decreased
  (c) corneal epithelial filaments
  (d) punctate epithelial erosions, ulceration
  (e) vital staining with Rose Bengal 1% (staining of interpalpebral devitalised cells and mucus)
  (f) Schirmer's tests:
    (i) type 1—wetting of Whatman no. 41 filter paper; basal secretion with topical anaesthesia, reflex without; normal basal—10–30 mm of wetting in 5 min
    (ii) type 2—measurement of basal secretion with nasal mucosal irritation
  (g) lysozyme assay: incubation of tears with bacteria (*Micrococcus lysodeikticus*) on agar plate for 24 hours; reduced activity in Sjögren's syndrome
  (h) tear osmolarity: normal (302 mosmol/l $\pm$ 6·3 mosmol/l); increased in aqueous deficiency (343 mosmol/l $\pm$ 32·3 mosmol/l)

CAUSES OF AQUEOUS DEFICIENCY

1 Idiopathic/age related
2 Primary and secondary Sjögren's syndrome

3 Inflammatory or infiltrative lesions, e.g. lymphoma, tuberculosis, sarcoidosis, syphilis
4 Riley–Day syndrome (familial dysautonomia) or congenital absence gland
5 Surgical removal of gland or irradiation
6 Sensory arc defect (trigeminal nerve defect)
7 Motor arc defect (facial nerve defect, cholinergic blockade)
8 Ductule scarring or destruction, e.g. removal of a lateral dermoid or dermolipoma
9 Medication, e.g. antihistamines, β-blockers, phenothiazines, contraceptive pill

MUCIN DEFICIENCY

1 Signs:
   (a) tear break up time: break up of fluorescein stained tear film in less than 10 seconds is abnormal
   (b) Bitot's spots: interpalpebral conjunctival foamy patches associated with severe vitamin A deficiency and xerophthalmia
2 Causes:
   (a) vitamin A deficiency
   (b) conjunctival cicatrisation resulting in goblet cell loss, e.g. chemical burns, Stevens–Johnson syndrome, cicatricial pemphigoid, trachoma

CAUSES OF AN ABNORMAL OILY LAYER

1 Blepharitis, often staphylococcal and compounding aqueous deficiency
2 Meibomianitis

MANAGEMENT OF DRY EYES

1 Artificial tears: if used very frequently consider preservative free tears
2 Lid hygiene with occasional courses of topical antibiotics
3 Mucolytic agents for filamentary keratitis
4 Supplemental vitamin A in xerophthalmia (topical retinoic acid, experimental)
5 Surgery to lid deformities or the insertion of nasal conchal grafts
6 Hydroxypropyl cellulose inserts
7 Punctal occlusion either temporary or permanent
8 Moist chamber goggles
9 Duct transposition rarely used
10 Stop exacerbating medication

EPIPHORA

1 Causes:
   (a) exclude eye disease:

(i) allergic, irritative, or infective conjunctivitis
(ii) trichiasis, distichiasis
(iii) corneal diseases
(b) dry eye with compensatory hypersecretion
(c) lacrimal pump failure, e.g. nerve VII palsy
(d) lid-globe incongruity such as ectropion
(e) obstruction of drainage system
(f) hypersecretion
2 Examination:
(a) exclude dry eye
(b) check punctal position and patency
(c) apply lacrimal sac pressure looking for reflux, i.e. mucocele
(d) nasal examination
(e) specific tests of patency:
(i) fluorescein disappearance test
(ii) taste test (saccharin/quinine)
(iii) Jones' primary test—staining of nasal swab after instillation of fluorescein in fornix
(iv) Jones' secondary test—if primary test is negative, irrigation of sac with saline; if staining of nasal swab occurs, dye was present in sac; if no staining lacrimal pump failure is the cause
(v) dacryoscintogram—instillation of technetium-99m (^{99m}Tc)
(vi) dacryocystogram—injection of Lipiodol; outlines drainage system
(vii) CT and MRI scans
(viii) probing—elucidates site of block; therapeutic manoeuvre to remove distal obstruction found in childhood

LACRIMAL DRAINAGE SYSTEM OBSTRUCTION

1 Causes:
(a) congenital:
(i) absence/atresia of the canaliculi and/or puncta
(ii) incomplete opening of the nasolacrimal duct
(iii) associated with facial anomalies
(b) senile: punctal stenosis or associated with chronic infection
(c) associated with ectropion and conjunctival cicatrisation
(d) trauma: physical or irradiation
(e) drug induced: practolol, idoxuridine, adrenaline, pilocarpine, and phospholine iodide
(f) inflammation: sarcoidosis, Wegner's granulomatosis, or pseudo-tumour
(g) infection:
(i) dacryocystitis—acute or chronic
(ii) canaliculitis—herpes simplex and zoster, *Actinomyces israelii*
(iii) sinusitis
(h) systemic disease, e.g. Paget's disease
(i) lacrimal sac tumours:
(i) primary, e.g. papilloma, squamous cell carcinoma

      (ii) secondary, e.g. basal cell carcinoma, lymphoma, sinus tumours
2 Treatment:
  (a) punctal:
      (i) dilatation ± one snip
      (ii) correct ectropion
      (iii) congenital—cut down or dacryocystorhinostomy (DCR) with retrograde intubation
  (b) canalicular:
      (i) within 8 mm of punctum—conjunctivodacryocystorhinostomy and Lester-Jones tubing
      (ii) more than 8 mm from punctum—canaliculodacryocystorhinostomy with intubation
      (iii) canaliculitis—commonly *Actinomyces israelii* (Gram positive anaerobic rod); irrigate with penicillin, canaliculotomy, and débridement
  (c) lacrimal sac:
      (i) acute dacryocystitis—painful swelling; treatment with antibiotics and drainage if necessary
      (ii) recurrent—dacryocystectomy first and then secondary Lester-Jones tubes; or DCR; epithelial fibrosis and scarring may cause obstruction of internal ostium and require stripping ± intubation
      (iii) chronic—results in obstruction and mucocele formation.
  (d) nasolacrimal duct obstruction:
      (i) congenital—failure of canalisation of inferior end of duct, resulting in recurrent conjunctivitis; treatment with lacrimal sac massage and antibiotics; probing after 1 year; rarely intubation, nasal turbinate infracture, or DCR
      (ii) acquired—mainstay of treatment is the DCR
      (iii) treat nasal pathology, e.g. polyps
  (e) lacrimal pump failure:
      (i) correct lid position and raise lateral canthus
      (ii) DCR

LACRIMAL GLAND INFLAMMATION

Causes:
1 Viral dacryoadenitis, e.g. mumps, glandular fever
2 Acute bacterial dacryoadenitis often secondary to conjunctivitis
3 Chronic bacterial, e.g. tuberculosis, syphilis
4 Inflammatory conditions, e.g. Sjögren's syndrome, sarcoidosis, Wegener's granulomatosis
5 Pseudotumour, reactive lymphoid hyperplasia, lymphoma

LACRIMAL GLAND TUMOURS

See chapter 2.

LACRIMAL SAC TUMOURS

1 Features:
  (a) rare
  (b) painless swelling
  (c) regurgitation of pus and blood via puncta
  (d) outlined with dacryocystogram
2 Histology:
  (a) transitional cell papilloma or carcinoma
  (b) squamous cell carcinoma (poorly differentiated)
  (c) adenocarcinoma

4
CONJUNCTIVA

Conjunctiva

1 Thin mucous membrane lining the conjunctival sac and continuous with the epithelium of the eyelids and cornea
2 Regions:
  (a) palpebral
      (i) marginal—extending from grey line to subtarsal groove
      (ii) tarsal—adherent to tarsal plates
      (iii) orbital—folded and loose, extending from peripheral borders of tarsus to fornices
  (b) forniceal: reflection reaching behind orbital rim extending behind globe equator forming fornices; receives attachments from the capsulopalpebral head of rectus muscles
  (c) bulbar: lining anterior sclera and pericorneal area
3 Semilunar fold: crescent shaped part of medial bulbar conjunctiva; narrow fold producing 2 mm cul de sac
4 Caruncle: at medial canthus; 3×5 mm; receives attachments from medical rectus; modified skin not conjunctiva

Conjunctival histology

1 Epithelium:
  (a) stratified non-keratinising epithelium:
      (i) basal epithelial cells include stem cells, melanocytes (numerous at limbus), and Langerhans' cells
      (ii) intermediate epithelial cells include wing cells
      (iii) goblet cells: numerous in lower fornix and plica
      (iv) second mucus secreting system's surface cells
      (v) extrinsic cells—includes macrophages, lymphocytes, granulocytes, and mast cells
  (b) regional variations:
      (i) marginal—transitional zone, squamous epithelium
      (ii) tarsal—2–4 layers of cells, columnar epithelium; rugged surface profile
      (iii) forniceal—4–8 layers, columnar
      (iv) bulbar—increasing number of intermediate layers, columnar, smooth profile

   (v) limbus—10–15 layers in basal fold, 2–3 on palisades of Vogt; squamous epithelium
   (vi) plica—8–10 layers numerous goblet cells, columnar
   (vii) caruncle—skin like; contains fine hairs, and sweat and sebaceous glands
2 Substantia propria: subepithelial fibrovascular loose connective tissue layers:
   (a) components:
      (i) blood vessels
      (ii) aqueous veins
      (iii) lymphatics—superficial and deep plexus
      (iv) nerves
      (v) glands—accessory lacrimal glands of Krause and Wolfring/Ciaccio
      (vi) non-striated muscle fibres
      (vii) cells—fibroblasts, macrophages, lymphocytes, plasma cells, mast cells, granulocytes, melanocytes
   (b) adenoidal layer:
      (i) develops by 3 months of age
      (ii) contains lymphoid follicles
      (iii) well developed in fornices
   (c) fibrous layer: deeper, connecting epithelium to Tenon's capsule

Blood supply of conjunctiva

1 Marginal arcade of eyelid: marginal conjunctiva
2 Peripheral arcade of eyelid: forniceal conjunctiva
3 Posterior conjunctival artery (branch of peripheral arcade) to within 4 mm of the limbus
4 Anterior conjunctival artery (branch of anterior ciliary artery): limbus; capillary arcades extend 1 mm into cornea
5 Veins: more numerous than arteries, but tend to follow them; drain mainly to superior and inferior ophthalmic veins
6 Capillaries: mainly non-fenestrated

Nerve supply of conjunctiva

1 Sensory:
   (a) branches of ophthalmic division of nerve V
   (b) branches of maxillary division of V (inferomedial)
2 Autonomic:
   (a) sympathetic: via plexus associated with branches of ophthalmic artery
   (b) parasympathetic: derived from the pterygopalatine ganglion

Lymphatic drainage of conjunctiva

1 Submandibular nodes drain:
   (a) medial $\frac{1}{3}$ of superior conjunctiva
   (b) medial $\frac{2}{3}$ of inferior conjunctiva

2 Preauricular nodes drain:
  (a) lateral $\frac{2}{3}$ of superior conjunctiva
  (b) lateral $\frac{1}{3}$ of inferior conjunctiva

Embryology

1 Epithelium: ectodermal origin; substantia propria—mesodermal; develops from 8 weeks
2 Plica semilunaris formed at same time as eyelids
3 Caruncle formed later by separation from lower lid at the time of canalicular formation

Conjunctival physiology

1 Tear production:
  (a) mucin (goblet cells)
  (b) aqueous (accessory lacrimal glands)
2 Supply oxygen directly to peripheral cornea when the eyes are open and to whole of the cornea when lids are closed
3 Defence mechanisms:
  (a) non-specific
      (i) from tear film (mucin clumping, aqueous phase mechanisms)
      (ii) intact epithelium acting as a physical barrier
      (iii) rich blood supply—good healing and delivery of immuno-competent cells
  (b) specific:
      (i) resident immunocompetent cells, e.g. mast cells, granulocytes, mucosa associated lymphoid tissue, and Langerhans' cells
      (ii) antibodies, e.g. secretory IgA
      (iii) recruitment of immunocompetent cells

CONJUNCTIVAL DISORDERS

1 Symptoms:
  (a) redness
  (b) stickiness/discharge
  (c) grittiness/foreign body sensation
  (d) photophobia
  (e) lacrimation
  (f) itching
2 Signs:
  (a) discharge:
      (i) serous (viral toxic)
      (ii) mucous (vernal)
      (iii) mucopurulent, purulent (bacterial, mycotic, vernal)
      (iv) purulent (bacterial)
      (v) pseudomembranous—strips off leaving intact epithelium (viral, gonococcal)
      (vi) membranous—strips off leaving ulcer
  (b) conjunctival "reaction":

      (i) hyperaemia
      (ii) oedema
      (iii) follicular reaction
      (iv) papillary reaction
      (v) haemorrhage
      (vi) granulomata
      (vii) scarring
      (viii) pigmentation

(c) associated corneal reaction
(d) associated lid (blepharitis, chalazia) and lacrimal (dacryocystitis) disease
(e) lymphadenopathy
(f) general examination, e.g. other mucous membranes, genitalia
(g) examination of sexual partners, children

3 Investigations:
(a) microscopy (conjunctival scraping)
  (i) Gram stain (bacteria and fungi)
  (ii) Giemsa stain (inflammatory cells, chlamydiae, and fungi)
  (iii) Papanicolaou's stain (viral inclusions)
  (iv) Ziehl–Neelsen stain (tuberculosis)
  (v) fluorescein labelled monoclonal antibody against invading organism, e.g. chlamydiae
(b) culture (conjunctival swabs):
  (i) blood agar (fungi and aerobic bacteria)
  (ii) thyoglycollate (anaerobes)
  (iii) chocolate agar (*Neisseria* and *Haemophilus* spp.)
  (iv) Sabouraud's agar (fungi)
  (v) brain–heart infusion (fungi)
  (vi) viral culture
(c) serial serum antibody measurement (to detect rising antibody titre)
(d) biopsy (bulbar conjunctiva, not fornix):
  (i) basement membrane disease
  (ii) possibly malignant lesions
  (iii) suspected sarcoid granulomata

Classification of conjunctivitis

1 According to cause:
(a) infective: bacterial, chlamydial, viral, or fungal
(b) chemical (toxic), trauma, and irradiation
(c) hypersensitivity:
  (i) drug allergy
  (ii) vernal conjunctivitis
  (iii) seasonal allergy (hay fever)
  (iv) giant papillary conjunctivitis
  (v) atopic keratoconjunctivitis
(d) drug induced, e.g. topical dipivefrine
2 According to exudate:
(a) serous
(b) mucoid

  (c) mucopurulent
  (d) purulent
  (e) pseudomembranous
  (f) membranous
  (g) ligneous
3 According to onset:
  (a) hyperacute
  (b) acute
  (c) chronic

Bacterial conjunctivitis

1 Hyperacute:
  (a) causes: *Neisseria gonorrheae* and *N. meningitidis*; can penetrate intact corneal epithelium
  (b) rapid onset (<24 hours)
  (c) copious purulent discharge
  (d) lid oedema, conjunctival chemosis, and severe injection
  (e) corneal infiltrates; ulcers may develop
2 Acute:
  (a) causes: *Haemophilus influenzae, H. aegyptius* (epidemic pinkeye) *Staphylococcus* spp.
  (b) conjunctival hyperaemia ± petechial haemorrhages
  (c) mild to moderate purulent discharge
3 Chronic:
  (a) causes: *Moraxella lacunata* (diplobacillus), staphylococci, chlamydiae
  (b) conjunctival hyperaemia, mucoid discharge
  (c) blepharitis (angular in moraxella infection)
  (d) marginal ulceration, phlyctenulosis
4 Membranous and pseudomembranous:
  (a) causes: *Corynebacterium diphtheriae*, β-haemolytic streptococci, *Streptococcus pneumoniae*
  (b) in chronic cases conjunctival scarring results
  (c) corneal infiltrates or ulceration may occur

Viral conjunctivitis

1 Adenoviral infections:
  (a) DNA viruses
  (b) 23 serotypes have been known to cause eye infections
  (c) mild to severe disease
  (d) bilateral follicular conjunctivitis with lymphadenopathy (often types 3, 4, 7, or 11)
  (e) pharyngoconjunctival fever (often types 3, 4, and 7); fever, pharyngitis, and keratitis in 30%
  (f) epidemic keratoconjunctivitis (often types 8, 10, and 19) + keratitis in 80%
  (g) keratitis more severe in epidemic keratoconjunctivitis:
       (i) diffuse punctate epithelial (week 1)
       (ii) focal epithelial (week 2)

    (iii) subepithelial (>week 2)
    (iv) grey epithelial (>week 2)
  (h) investigations:
      (i) HeLa/HEK/Hep-2 cell culture detection/typing using mono-
          clonal antibody techniques
      (ii) rising serum antibody titres
  (i) treatment:
      (i) supportive as self limiting in 2–3 weeks
      (ii) personal hygiene to prevent spread
      (iii) topical steroids for severe keratitis (may prolong course of
          infiltrates)
      (iv) antibiotics to prevent secondary infection—occurs in 10%
2 Herpes simplex virus and herpes zoster virus:
  (a) DNA viruses
  (b) follicular conjunctivitis with or without corneal lesions
  (c) primary or recurrent
3 Myxoviruses:
  (a) RNA viruses
  (b) measles:
      (i) acute catarrhal conjunctivitis
      (ii) corneal erosions
      (iii) Koplick's spots on caruncle
4 Paramyxoviruses:
  (a) RNA viruses
  (b) mumps:
      (i) painful dacryoadenitis
      (ii) follicular conjunctivitis
      (iii) keratitis
  (c) Newcastle disease:
      (i) unilateral conjunctivitis
      (ii) pneumonitis (spread from fowl)
5 Picornaviruses (e.g. Enterovirus 70):
  (a) RNA viruses
  (b) acute haemorrhagic conjunctivitis
  (c) rapid onset, bilateral
6 Molluscum contagiosum (pox virus) and verruca vulgaris (human
  papilloma virus):
  (a) chronic follicular conjunctivitis
  (b) associated lid lesions
  (c) superficial keratitis
  (d) pannus

Chlamydial infections

1 Adult inclusion conjunctivitis:
  (a) causes:
      (i) serovars D–K cause inclusion conjunctivitis (adult [AIC] and
          neonatal [NIC])
      (ii) intracellular organism transmitted sexually (urethritis cervici-
          tis)

    (b) features:
- (i) bilateral, acute, mucopurulent
- (ii) follicular with papillae on upper tarsal conjunctiva
- (iii) preauricular lymphadenopathy
- (iv) chronic course if untreated
- (v) keratitis mainly in superior cornea—epithelial, subepithelial nummular lesions, marginal infiltrates, and micropannus.

    (c) investigations:
- (i) basophilic cytoplasmic inclusion bodies (Halberstaedter–Prowazek) on Giemsa staining
- (ii) monoclonal antibody techniques such as ELISA (enzyme linked immunosorbent assay) and fluorescein linked antibodies

    (d) management:
- (i) investigation of genitourinary system
- (ii) systemic and topical tetracycline or erythromycin for 3–6 weeks
- (iii) investigation of sexual contacts

2 Neonatal inclusion conjunctivitis:

    (a) causes:
- (i) serovars D–K
- (ii) infection transmitted to child during vaginal delivery

    (b) features:
- (i) onset 5–14 days
- (ii) acute, mucopurulent, or purulent
- (iii) papillary; no follicles until 3 months of age
- (iv) superior pannus, conjunctival scarring
- (v) systemic infection may be present—pneumonitis, otitis, rhinitis, gastritis

    (c) management:
- (i) swabs—ocular, rectal, throat, ear
- (ii) investigation of mother and sexual contacts
- (iii) topical tetracycline and systemic erythromycin
- (iv) prophylactic topical treatment for 1 week when born to an infected mother

3 Trachoma:

    (a) the world's second major blinding condition; 6–9 million people blind (<3/60) from trachoma (1984 WHO estimate).

    (b) cause: serovars A, B, and C

    (c) infection–reinfection cycle through person to person contact or by flies

    (d) lack of immunity to infecting agent

    (e) predominantly women and children affected

    (f) classification:
- (i) TF: trachomatous inflammation—follicular; >5 follicles of >0·5 mm on upper tarsus
- (ii) TI: trachomatous inflammation—intense; inflammatory thickening obscuring >50% of large deep tarsal vessels
- (iii) TS: trachomatous (conjunctival) cicatrisation—visible white lines, bands, or sheets of fibrosis

    (iv) TT: trachomatous trichiasis—at least 1 eyelash or evidence of recent removal

    (v) CO: corneal opacity—obscuring at least part of pupil margin; causing vision < 6/18

(g) corneal changes:
    (i) epithelial keratitis
    (ii) infiltrates
    (iii) superior superficial pannus
    (iv) Herbert's pits (cicatrised limbal follicles)
    (v) secondary corneal infections

(h) investigations:
    (i) basophilic inclusion bodies in conjunctival scrapings during active disease
    (ii) fluorescent monoclonal antibody staining

(i) management:
    (i) during active disease; systemic and topical antibiotics (tetracycline or erythromycin)
    (ii) lid surgery for eyelid and eyelash malposition
    (iii) management of dry eyes
    (iv) public health measures—hand and face washing, topical antibiotics (tetracycline or erythromycin), or annual erythromycin

Ophthalmia neonatorum

1 Conjunctivitis within first month of life
2 Notifiable disease in the UK
3 Types:
    (a) chemical, e.g. silver nitrate; occurs within 24 hours of instillation
    (b) gonococcal:
        (i) 2–4 days
        (ii) hyperacute, purulent, haemorrhagic conjunctivitis
        (iii) corneal ulceration, perforation
        (iv) management—urgent Gram stain looking for Gram negative intracellular diplococci; topical and systemic antibiotics
    (c) staphylococcal: 4–5 days
    (d) *Haemophilus* spp.: 4–5 days
    (e) herpes simplex:
        (i) 5–7 days
        (ii) type 2 virus
        (iii) non-purulent blepharoconjunctivitis
        (iv) keratitis
        (v) management—intravenous acyclovir, parental investigations
    (f) chlamydial:
        (i) 5–14 days
        (ii) most common cause

Ligneous conjunctivitis

1 Features:
    (a) rare, usually bilateral

    (b) affects young children
    (c) acute onset, chronic recurrent course
    (d) possibly related to excessive abnormal mucus
2 Pathology:
    (a) pseudomembrane with development of large amounts of granulation tissue
    (b) late compaction and invasion of tissue by plasma cells and eosinophils
3 Management:
    (a) usually undergoes spontaneous resolution
    (b) may require surgical excision of large masses; intensive postoperative topical heparin

Parinaud's oculoglandular syndrome

1 Features:
    (a) unilateral mucopurulent discharge
    (b) conjunctival granulomata
    (c) follicles with necrosis and ulceration
    (d) ipsilateral lymphadenopathy
    (e) fever and malaise
2 Causes:
    (a) cat scratch fever
    (b) oculoglandular tularaemia
    (c) sporotrichosis
    (d) tuberculosis
    (e) syphilis
    (f) coccidioidomycosis
    (g) lymphogranuloma venereum

(Seasonal) allergic conjunctivitis

1 Features:
    (a) type I hypersensitivity; commonly to pollens
    (b) bilateral, acute, and recurrent
    (c) lacrimation, chemosis, rhinitis
2 Management:
    (a) avoidance of allergens
    (b) topical sodium cromoglycate
    (c) topical or systemic antihistamines
    (d) topical steroids
    (e) desensitisation

Vernal keratoconjunctivitis (VKC)

1 Features:
    (a) recurrent, bilateral inflammation
    (b) especially spring and summer
    (c) more common in the tropics
    (d) more common in children and young adults especially males
    (e) burnout occurs in about 10 years

(f) family/personal history of atopy is common
2 Symptoms:
  (a) itching, lacrimation, photophobia, and grittiness
  (b) stringy mucous discharge
  (c) itchy skin
3 Signs:
  (a) limbal:
    (i) limbal follicles
    (ii) Trantas' dots (eosinophils clumped at apex of follicles)
  (b) palpebral:
    (i) cobblestone papillae of varying size and shape
    (ii) ptosis in severe cases
  (c) keratitis:
    (i) punctate epithelial keratitis (superior)
    (ii) epithelial macroerosions
    (iii) plaque (shield ulcer); non-wetting ulcer, poor healing
    (iv) subepithelial scarring
    (v) pseudogerontoxon—"Cupid's bow" appearance
  (d) ptosis
4 Pathology:
  (a) flat topped giant papillae (cobblestones)
  (b) hypertrophy of adenoidal layers
  (c) mast cell (mainly degranulated) cell infiltrate
  (d) epithelial downgrowth
  (e) goblet cell proliferation
  (f) fibrosis, hyaline degeneration
  (g) alkaline tears
  (h) eosinophilia
  (i) raised tear and serum IgE
5 Treatment:
  (a) mast cell stabilisers, e.g. topical sodium cromoglycate drops
  (b) lubricants
  (c) mucolytic agents
  (d) topical steroids
  (e) débridement of plaques
  (f) oral antihistamines

Atopic keratoconjunctivitis

1 Features:
  (a) ocular manifestation of atopy
  (b) chronic, bilateral, external, ocular inflammation with atopic dermatitis
  (c) most common in young adults with a family history of atopy
  (d) may not resolve for 50 years
2 Symptoms and signs:
  (a) irritation, itching, and stringy discharge
  (b) lid dermatitis and staphylococcal blepharitis
  (c) inferior conjunctiva involved
  (d) conjunctival shrinkage and symblepharon

(e) corneal pannus and punctate keratopathy
(f) cataract and keratoconus
3 Treatment: similar to vernal keratoconjunctivitis

Giant papillary conjunctivitis (GPC)

1 Features:
  (a) giant papillae (>3 mm diameter) affecting upper tarsal conjunctiva
  (b) irritation, itching, and stringy discharge
2 Causes:
  (a) contact lens wear (particularly soft lenses)
  (b) ocular prosthesis
  (c) protruding corneal sutures

Toxic conjunctivitis

1 Features:
  (a) chronic follicular conjunctivitis affecting mainly inferior conjunctiva
  (b) conjunctival cicatrisation with prolonged topical medication
  (c) punctate or ulcerative keratitis
2 Causes:
  (a) preservatives in eyedrops
  (b) topical treatments:
      (i) antibiotics, e.g. neomycin, gentamicin
      (ii) glaucoma medications, e.g. pilocarpine, dipivefrine
      (iii) atropine
  (c) blepharitis (meibomian secretions)
  (d) contact lens solutions
3 Treatment:
  (a) avoidance of irritant
  (b) trial of preservative free drops

Phlyctenulosis

1 Features:
  (a) usually affects children
  (b) unilateral bulbar conjunctival nodules (0·5–3 mm)
  (c) often at limbus
2 Causes: type IV sensitivity to staphylococci (most common) or *Mycobacterium tuberculosis*
3 Management:
  (a) treatment of primary condition
  (b) topical steroids and antibiotics

Mucous membrane pemphigoid   *predominantly mm – OCP, skin – Bullous Pemph*

1 Features:
  (a) autoimmune disease with deposition of immunoglobulins and complement in the basement membrane; associated with HLA-B12 (and HLA-DQw7)

    (b) onset in 6th to 7th decade
    (c) F:M = 2:1
    (d) skin involvement:
        (i) recurrent vesicobullous lesions in inguinal areas and extremities
        (ii) scarring lesions over scalp and face (80%)
    (e) mucous membrane involvement:
        (i) gingivae (90%)
        (ii) buccal (25–30%)
        (iii) pharynx, larynx, oesophagus, anus, and vagina
    (f) ocular:
        (i) bilateral, relentless progression
        (ii) non-specific hyperaemia, papillary conjunctivitis, pseudomembranes
        (iii) subconjunctival fibrosis (fornix shrinkage) and symblepharon
        (iv) aqueous (sicca) and mucus (xerosis) tear deficiency
        (v) corneal exposure, opacification, and vascularisation
        (vi) secondary bacterial infection
2 Histology:
    (a) epithelial thinning
    (b) loss of goblet cells
    (c) keratinisation
    (d) subepithelial inflammation and fibrosis
    (e) antibasement membrane antibody on immunofluorescent staining
3 Treatment:
    (a) lubricants, punctal occlusion, moist chamber goggles
    (b) antibiotics
    (c) contact lens
    (d) treatment of trichiasis and entropion
        (eyelid surgery may exacerbate condition)
    (e) systemic corticosteroids, immunosuppressive agents, or dapsone
    (f) keratoprostheses

Stevens–Johnson syndrome

1 Features:
    (a) affects young people.
    (b) precipitated by infections or drugs
    (c) associated with HLA-Bw44
2 Characterised by:
    (a) skin lesions (erythema multiforme):
        (i) vesicles and bullae
        (ii) target lesions
        (iii) extensor surfaces
    (b) mucous membranes:
        (i) acute ulceration, and late scarring and strictures
        (ii) oral, oesophageal, and genitourinary membranes affected
    (c) acute ocular findings:
        (i) lid swelling, ulceration, and crusting
        (ii) pseudomembranous or membranous conjunctivitis

(iii) anterior uveitis
(d) late ocular findings:
    (i) subepithelial fibrosis, shrinkage, and symblepharon
    (ii) trichiasis, entropion, and lagophthalmos
    (iii) dry eye syndrome caused by fibrosis of lacrimal gland ducts and loss of goblet cells, resulting in keratinisation
    (iv) corneal exposure, opacification, pannus
    (v) visual loss resulting from corneal scarring
(e) general:
    (i) arthralgia
    (ii) fever
    (iii) sore throat
    (iv) malaise

3 Causes:
(a) post infection (bacteria, *Mycoplasma pneumoniae*, herpes simplex virus)
(b) drugs:
    (i) sulphonamides; 25% recurrence on re-exposure
    (ii) other antibiotics, e.g. tetracyclines and penicillin
    (iii) non-steroidal anti-inflammatory drugs (NSAIDs)
    (iv) barbiturates

4 Histopathology (conjunctiva):
(a) early:
    (i) epithelial thinning
    (ii) fibrinous exudate
    (iii) stromal lymphocytic infiltrate
    (iv) immunoglobulin and complement deposited at dermal–epidermal junction
(b) late:
    (i) patchy epidermalisation (rete pegs, prickle cells, epithelial thickening, and keratinisation)
    (ii) subepithelial fibrosis

5 Management:
(a) remove causative agents
(b) lubricants
(c) steroids (oral and topical)
(d) symblepharon lysis
(e) topical antibiotics to prevent secondary infection
(f) lid and conjunctival surgery to treat trichiasis, entropion, and corneal exposure
(g) topical retinoic acid (to reduce keratinisation after the active inflammation has resolved)

Superior limbic keratoconjunctivitis

1 Affects mainly middle aged women
2 Symptoms:
(a) photophobia and tearing
(b) foreign body sensation and pain
(c) recurrent condition despite treatment

3 Associations:
  (a) dysthyroid eye disease
  (b) following intraocular surgery
  (c) contact lens wear
4 Features:
  (a) chronic, recurrent inflammation of the superior limbus (50% bilateral)
  (b) superior tarsal papillary hypertrophy
  (c) bulbar conjunctival injection
  (d) limbitis
  (e) filamentary keratitis (30%)
  (f) Rose Bengal staining of superior cornea, limbus, and bulbar conjunctiva
5 Management:
  (a) lubricants
  (b) acetylcysteine drops
  (c) soft contact lens
  (d) recession or resection of superior bulbar conjunctiva
  (e) check thyroid status
  (f) no relief with either topical antibiotics or steroids

Degenerations

1 Lithiasis: concretions; resulting from prolonged conjunctivitis
2 Pinguecula:
  (a) yellow–white perilimbal plaques in interpalpebral area
  (b) may be caused by chronic actinic exposure
  (c) histology:
      (i) epithelial thinning
      (ii) elastoid stromal degeneration
3 Pterygium:
  (a) wing shaped fibrovascular overgrowth onto cornea in interpalpebral space, usually nasally
  (b) may be related to chronic actinic exposure
  (c) histology:
      (i) epithelial thinning
      (ii) elastoid degeneration
      (iii) fragmentation of Bowman's membrane
      (iv) iron deposition line, anterior to head of pterygium (Stocker's line)
  (d) indications for treatment:
      (i) cosmetic
      (ii) visual axis threatened
      (iii) astigmatism
  (e) treatments:
      (i) excision leaving bare sclera
      (ii) lamellar corneal graft
      (iii) conjunctival autograft
      (iv) excision with β-radiation, mitomycin, or thiotepa to prevent recurrences

"Cystic" conjunctival lesions

1 Simple cysts (serous)
2 Implantation cysts:
   (a) surgical
   (b) traumatic
3 Granulomata:
   (a) retained foreign body
   (b) suture material
4 Dermoids:
   (a) congenitally displaced embryonic epithelium
   (b) usually present at and adherent to the limbus (inferotemporal)
   (c) consists of keratinising dermal tissue with dermal appendages
   (d) Goldenhar's syndrome:
       (i) bilateral limbal dermoids
       (ii) preauricular skin tags
       (iii) aural fistulae, vertebral anomalies
       (iv) facial and widespread neuromuscular and skeletal anomalies

Conjunctival vascular anomalies

1 Lymphangiectasia: dilated lymph channels
2 Telangiectasia:
   (a) ataxia–telangiectasia (Louis–Bar syndrome)
   (b) Osler–Weber–Rendu syndrome
   (c) Sturge–Weber syndrome
   (d) extracranial/intracranial fistula
   (e) irradiation
   (f) mustard gas

Non-pigmented conjunctival lesions (A: epithelial)

1 Papilloma:
   (a) viral: younger ages group, may be multiple; no malignant potential; human papilloma virus (HPV) can be isolated
   (b) non-viral: sessile lesions in older individuals; potential for malignant transformation
   (c) both types require excision with cryotherapy to base
2 Actinic keratoses (dyskeratosis, leukoplasia):
   (a) premalignant epithelial hyperplasia
   (b) keratinisation
   (c) elastoid degeneration of the stroma with or without inflammation
3 Xeroderma pigmentosa:
   (a) usually autosomal recessive
   (b) UV light induced premalignant lesions
4 Conjunctival intraepithelial dysplasia (CID):
   (a) more common over 60 years of age
   (b) men > women
   (c) interpalpebral, perilimbal, raised, reddish–grey, and vascularised lesion
   (d) slow growing and may invade the cornea
   (e) malignant potential

   (f) risk factors: UV light, petroleum, smoking, and HPV infection
   (g) histopathology:
      (i) characterised by loss of normal progression of cell maturation
      (ii) proliferation of basal cells
      (iii) loss of cellular polarity
      (iv) hyperchromatic nuclei
      (v) mitotic activity
      (vi) basement membrane intact
   (h) management: excision biopsy ± cryotherapy
5 Squamous cell carcinoma:
   (a) macroscopically similar to CID but stromal invasion has occurred
   (b) local and distant spread
   (c) histopathology:
      (i) hyperkeratosis, dyskeratosis, and acanthosis
      (ii) stromal invasion
   (d) management:
      (i) excision biopsy avoiding damage to Bowman's membrane
      (ii) cryotherapy
      (iii) radiotherapy
      (iv) prognosis good if no metastatic spread, but high focal recurrence rate
6 Mucoepidermoid and spindle cell carcinoma:
   (a) rare variants of squamous cell carcinoma
   (b) more aggressive
   (c) ocular invasion may occur

Non-pigmented conjunctival lesions (A: non-epithelial)

1 Conjunctival lymphoma:
   (a) classification (MALT = mucosa associated lymphoid tissue):
      (i) benign MALT hyperplasia
      (ii) MALT lymphoma
      (iii) non-MALT lymphoma (non-Hodgkin's)
   (b) features:
      (i) variable appearance, classically diffuse salmon pink infiltrates
      (ii) can be confused with GPC or severe follicular conjunctivitis
      (iii) may invade orbit
   (c) pathology:
      (i) MALT lymphoma—B cell, low grade, good prognosis
      (ii) non-MALT lymphoma—follicular or non-follicular, poor prognosis
   (d) management:
      (i) MALT lymphoma—biopsy and radiotherapy
      (ii) non-MALT lymphoma—biopsy, systemic evaluation, systemic chemotherapy
2 Kaposi's sarcoma:
   (a) tumour of lymphatic endothelial cells
   (b) increasing incidence, especially in patients with AIDS
   (c) bluish–red vascular lesion, nodular or diffuse
   (d) responds well to radiotherapy

3 Other tumours:
  (a) rare
  (b) benign or malignant
  (c) may originate from glandular tissue, connective tissue, vascular tissue, or peripheral nerves

Pigmented conjunctival lesions

1 Pseudopigmented lesions:
  (a) blue sclera, e.g. in osteogenesis imperfecta, Ehlers–Danlos, and Marfan's syndromes
  (b) scleromalacia perforans
  (c) staphylomas
2 Exogenous causes of pigmentation:
  (a) argyria
  (b) mascara
  (c) adrenochromes
3 Endogenous causes of pigmentation:
  (a) Addison's disease
  (b) Nelson's syndrome
  (c) alkaptonuria:
      (i) autosomal recessive
      (ii) absence of homogentisic acid oxidase (dark urine reducing Benedict's reagent)
  (d) jaundice
  (e) around perforating arteries
4 Epithelial melanosis:
  (a) racial (perilimbal)
  (b) primary acquired melanosis (PAM):
      (i) middle age
      (ii) patchy, flat pigmentation that may advance or regress with time
      (iii) premalignant; presence of atypia on histology indicated a higher chance of malignant transformation
  (c) secondary:
      (i) exposure
      (ii) ectropion
      (iii) trachoma
      (iv) onchocerciasis
5 Subepithelial melanosis:
  (a) congenital
  (b) associated with eyelid pigmentation (naevus of Ota); these cases may be associated with choroidal melanoma, uveitis, and glaucoma
6 Naevi:
  (a) features:
      (i) common; appear in childhood or at puberty
      (ii) single, sharply demarcated, flat, or elevated
      (iii) usually brown or black but 30% amelanotic
      (iv) may increase at puberty or during pregnancy

(v) no deep attachments—can be moved with cotton tipped applicator

(vi) may contain small cysts

(vii) malignant transition rare

(b) treatment: excision for cosmesis, irritation, or if malignant change suspected

(c) histology:

(i) similar features to cutaneous naevi, i.e. junctional, sub-epithelial, or compound

(ii) in addition, solid and cystic epithelial inclusions derived from surface epithelium may occur

7 Malignant melanoma:

(a) may arise *de novo*, in PAM, or in a naevus

(b) mainly affects white European adults

(c) features:

(i) diffuse or nodular

(ii) unifocal or multifocal

(iii) melanotic or amelanotic

(iv) dilated feeder vessel may be present

(d) poor prognostic factors:

(i) thickness >1–2 mm

(ii) forniceal or palpebral location (late presentation)

(iii) epithelioid cell type

(iv) lymphatic invasion and metastasis

(e) management:

(i) periodic observation

(ii) excision if shows >0·5 mm elevation

(iii) cryotherapy

(iv) excision with cryotherapy

(v) radiotherapy (e.g. if excision incomplete)

(vi) exenteration

Chemical injury

1 Acid burn:

(a) limited injury

(b) proteins denatured

2 Alkali burn:

(a) saponification of lipid ∴ damaging Cell membrane

(b) deep ocular penetration with potentially severe damage and ischaemia

(c) complications:

(i) symblepharon

(ii) xerosis

(iii) corneal ulceration, failure of epithelialisation, stromal ulceration, and stromal melt; late vascularisation

(iv) uveitis

(v) cataract

(vi) secondary glaucoma

(vii) phthisis

(d) treatment:
  - (i) copious irrigation
  - (ii) mydriasis and cycloplegia
  - (iii) analgesia
  - (iv) steroids (week 1)
  - (v) sodium ascorbate 10% drops
  - (vi) collagenase inhibitors
  - (vii) lubricants
  - (viii) symblepharon lysis and prevention, e.g. contact lens
  - (ix) eyelid surgery
  - (x) keratoplasty later (poor results)

Drugs causing cicatricial conjunctival disease

1 Systemic:
  (a) practolol (oculomucocutaneous syndrome)
2 Topical:
  (a) chronic use of anti-glaucoma drugs:
    - (i) miotics (pilocarpine, ecothiopate iodide)
    - (ii) sympathomimetics (adrenaline, dipivefrine)
    - (iii) ?β-blockers
    - (iv) ?role of preservatives
  (b) antiviral agents:
    - (i) trifluorothymidine (F_3T)
    - (ii) idoxuridine

5
CORNEA AND SCLERA

CORNEA

1 Dimensions:
   (a) average horizontal diameter 11·5 mm
   (b) thickness: 1 mm peripherally, 0·5 mm centrally
   (c) radius of curvature: anterior surface 7·8 mm, posterior surface 6·6 mm
2 Histology:
   (a) epithelium: 5–6 cells deep, non-keratinising, stratified, squamous; zona occludens and microvilli at surface; regenerates
   (b) Bowman's layer: anterior condensation of substantia propria; scars with trauma
   (c) substantia propria (stroma): avascular network of interlacing collagen fibrils, scattered keratocytes, mucopolysaccharide, and glycoprotein ground substance; corneal nerves
   (d) Descemet's membrane: strong collagenous layer; resistant to chemicals and infective agents; readily regenerates
   (e) endothelium: polygonal cell monolayer; cells cannot regenerate
3 Embryology:
   (a) epithelium derived from surface ectoderm
   (b) rest derived from mesenchyme

Physiology

1 Functions:
   (a) light refraction; cornea 43 D (versus 15 D from lens *in situ*)
   (b) reduction of oblique and spherical optical aberrations (caused by aplanatic surface)
   (c) protection against physical, chemical, and infective agents
   (d) transmission of light in 400–700 nm wavelength band
2 Composition:
   (a) 78% water
   (b) 4% mucopolysaccharides
   (c) 18% collagen
3 Thickness affected by:
   (a) age
   (b) osmolarity of tears

    (c) intraocular pressure
    (d) integrity of epithelium and endothelium
    (e) drugs
    (f) temperature
    (g) disease
4 Transparency resulting from:
    (a) relative dehydration
    (b) absence of blood vessels and pigments
    (c) regular arrangement of stromal layers and collagen fibrils
    (d) consistent refractive index of all layers (1·376)
5 Metabolism:
    (a) mostly in endothelium, epithelium, and stromal keratocytes
    (b) preferably aerobic (can survive 7 hours anaerobically)
    (c) oxygen: mostly derived from tear film; some from limbal capillaries (oxygen gradient from tears to the aqueous)
    (d) glucose: 90% derived from aqueous, 10% from limbal capillaries
6 Permeability:
    (a) lipid rich hydrophobic epithelium and endothelium; good permeability to water and lipids, poor to salts; hydrophilic stroma
    (b) relative dehydration caused by integrity of hydrophobic epithelium and endothelium
    (c) osmotic gradient (aqueous and tears are hypertonic)

SCLERA

1 Tough fibrous envelope composed of collagen and elastic fibres
2 Thickness:
    (a) 1 mm posteriorly
    (b) 0·33 mm beneath recti
    (c) 0·66 mm at insertion of recti
3 Radius of curvature of 12 mm
4 Three ill defined layers:
    (a) episclera
    (b) sclera proper
    (c) lamina fusca
5 Pierced by:
    (a) optic nerve via lamina cribrosa
    (b) vortex veins
    (c) posterior ciliary nerves and vessels
    (d) anterior ciliary arteries
    (e) episcleral veins
6 Embryology: derived from mesenchyme

CONGENITAL CORNEAL DISEASE

1 Microcornea:
    (a) bilateral
    (b) <10 mm horizontal diameter

    (c) associated shallow anterior chamber and narrow angle; angle closure glaucoma
2 Megalocornea:
    (a) bilateral horizontal diameter >13 mm (> 12 mm in neonates)
    (b) no associated glaucoma
    (c) non-progressive
    (d) posterior subcapsular cataract occurs
3 Sclerocornea:
    (a) autosomal recessive or dominant
    (b) non-inflammatory vascularised peripheral corneal opacification
    (c) non-progressive
    (d) associations:
        (i) cornea plana
        (ii) aniridia
        (iii) mesodermal dysgenesis
        (iv) microphthalmos
4 Epibulbar dermoids: limbal or central

Anterior corneal dystrophies

1 Cogan's:
    (a) microcystic, map, dot, or fingerprint appearance
    (b) often asymptomatic
    (c) can cause recurrent erosions
    (d) presents in fourth decade
    (e) vision unaffected unless frank epithelial breakdown
    (f) symptomatic treatment or, recently, excimer laser phototherapeutic keratectomy (PTK)
2 Reis–Bückler's:
    (a) autosomal dominant
    (b) most common dystrophy
    (c) typical central honeycomb appearance with progressive scarring of Bowman's membrane
    (d) affects epithelium, Bowman's membrane, and anterior stroma
    (e) presents in childhood with recurrent erosions
    (f) vision impaired by teens
    (g) symptomatic treatment; eventually requires graft or PTK
3 Meesmann's:
    (a) autosomal dominant; onset in infancy
    (b) rare
    (c) clear epithelial microcysts
    (d) vision unaffected
    (e) periodic acid–Schiff (PAS) positive staining
    (f) symptomatic treatment

Stromal corneal dystrophies

1 Lattice:
    (a) autosomal dominant
    (b) appearance of branching crisscrossed lines of amyloid
    (c) initially anterior stroma, deeper later

    (d) presents in childhood/teens; recurrent erosions

    (e) vision impaired by 30s—especially glare which is disabling

    (f) localised deposits of amyloid (stains with PAS and Congo red, exhibits birefringence)

    (g) eventually requires corneal grafting

    (h) may recur in graft 4–5 years after grafting

2 Macular:

    (a) autosomal recessive

    (b) most severe corneal dystrophy

    (c) all layers affected (initially superficial)

    (d) greyish macular lesions, initially central

    (e) recurrent erosions in childhood; vision impaired by 30s—disability resulting from glare

    (f) mucopolysaccharide deposition in keratocytes and stroma (stains with colloidal iron and Alcian blue)

    (g) eventually requires corneal grafting

    (h) recurrence can occur in graft

3 Granular:

    (a) autosomal dominant

    (b) relatively mild

    (c) central, crumb like opacities

    (d) initially anterior stroma; deeper later

    (e) present in teens with photophobia or abnormal appearance (recurrent erosions are rare)

    (f) vision often normal or only impaired in 40s—disability resulting from glare

    (g) local deposits of abnormal proteins (stains with Masson's trichrome)

    (h) occasionally needs full thickness graft (recurrence is unusual)

Endothelial corneal dystrophies

1 Fuchs':

    (a) weak familial tendency (no specific inheritance)

    (b) relatively common

    (c) 40–70 year age group; more common in women

    (d) excrescences on Descemet's membrane with abnormal endothelial cell morphology

    (e) initially axial and asymptomatic—pachymetry aids diagnosis (corneal thickness greatest in morning)

    (f) later endothelial decompensation and bullous keratopathy; visual acuity worse on waking

    (g) treat with hyperosmotic agents, bandage contact lens

    (h) eventually requires full thickness graft

2 Posterior polymorphous:

    (a) autosomal dominant

    (b) asymmetrical, vesicle like lesions in Descemet's membrane, variable morphology (can have a "tramline" appearance)

    (c) abnormal collagenous membrane is secreted by the endothelium

    (d) usually asymptomatic; evident from teens onwards

(e) occasionally associated with iridoschisis, band keratopathy, glaucoma

(f) no treatment required

Ectatic corneal dystrophies

1 Keratoconus:
   (a) unknown aetiology; occasionally familial; onset in teens
   (b) incidence 1:20 000
   (c) thinning and bowing forward of inferior paracentral cornea
   (d) progressive blurring of vision as a result of irregular astigmatism and compound myopic astigmatism
   (e) other signs:
        (i) Munson's sign (bulging of the lower lid when the patient looks down)
        (ii) Fleischer's ring (iron depositions in basal epithelium cells)
        (iii) Vogt's lines (vertical stromal striae)
        (iv) central scarring
        (v) prominent corneal nerves
        (vi) oil drop sign—altered retinoscopic or ophthalmoscopic light reflex
   (f) acute hydrops can occur
   (g) treat initially with hard contact lens; full thickness graft required in about 20% of cases
   (h) associations:
        (i) atopy
        (ii) Down's syndrome (eye rubbing may be a factor)
        (iii) Turner's syndrome
        (iv) Marfan's syndrome
        (v) Ehlers–Danlos syndrome
        (vi) aniridia
        (vii) retinitis pigmentosa
        (viii) ectopia lentis
        (ix) microcornea
        (x) non-specific systemic collagen abnormalities
2 Posterior keratoconus:
   (a) rare, non-progressive
   (b) posterior corneal surface has variable sized excavations with no associated scarring
3 Keratoglobus:
   (a) rare
   (b) unknown aetiology
   (c) thinning of entire cornea
   (d) irregular astigmatism
   (e) treatment similar to keratoconus
4 Pellucid marginal degeneration:
   (a) rare
   (b) peripheral corneal thinning
   (c) irregular astigmatism
   (d) occasional hydrops

CORNEAL DEGENERATIONS

1 Band shaped keratopathy:
  (a) extracellular deposition of calcium and hydroxyapatite in basement membrane, Bowman's layer, and superficial stroma
  (b) in the interpalpebral zone
  (c) Swiss cheese appearance (possibly as a result of perforation by corneal nerves)
  (d) associated with chronic anterior uveitis (especially juvenile chronic arthritis), hypercalcaemia, phthisis
  (e) treatment:
    (i) bandage contact lens
    (ii) superficial keratectomy (including excimer laser PTK)
    (iii) topical EDTA
    (iv) lamellar grafting
2 Saltzmann's nodular degeneration:
  (a) superficial bluish-white nodules
  (b) hyaline deposits in Bowman's membrane
  (c) vision may be unaffected
  (d) can result from chronic inflammatory conditions such as syphilitic keratitis, phlyctenular keratitis, trachoma, viral keratitis
  (e) associated with aniridia
  (f) eventually may need superficial keratectomy
3 Spheroid degeneration (Labrador keratopathy):
  (a) spherical extracellular deposits of eosinophilic material (degenerative collagen)
  (b) in subepithelial cornea (and conjunctiva)
  (c) related to UV irradiation
  (d) may require graft
4 Lipid keratopathy:
  (a) extracellular deposition of lipid
  (b) adjacent to areas of corneal vascularisation (e.g. post HSV keratitis)

CORNEAL INFECTIONS

Bacterial corneal infections
1 Clinical presentations:
  (a) keratitis
  (b) keratoconjunctivitis
  (c) hypopyon ulcer
2 Predisposing factors:
  (a) adnexal infection
  (b) entropion
  (c) exposure
  (d) dry eyes
  (e) contact lens wear
  (f) other corneal disease, e.g. bullous keratopathy

3 Types:
  (a) *Staphylococcus aureus/Streptococcus pneumoniae* produce yellowish opaque, oval stromal infection
  (b) *Pseudomonas aeruginosa* produces an irregular ulcer, diffuse necrosis, semiopaque surrounding cornea, rapid progression; may perforate.
  (c) Enterobacteriaceae cause shallow ulcers, grey–white suppuration, and diffuse stromal opacity
  (d) *Neisseria gonorrhoeae, N. menigitidis,* and *Corynebacterium diphtheriae* are unusual causes; associated with purulent conjunctivitis; may perforate

Chlamydia trachomatis
1 Adult inclusion conjunctivitis (TRIC):
  (a) serotypes D–K
  (b) superficial punctate keratitis in 75%
2 Trachoma:
  (a) serotype A, B, or C
  (b) superficial keratitis in acute stage
  (c) later superior pannus formation

Adenovirus

1 Common, highly infectious
2 Superficial punctate erosions
3 Subepithelial, nummular, circular, "coin like" opacities
4 Follicular conjunctivitis
5 Topical steroids alleviate the keratitis

Other viral causes of follicular conjunctivitis

1 Myxoviruses (measles)
2 Paramyxoviruses (mumps)
3 Molluscum contagiosum
4 Epstein–Barr virus (infectious mononucleosis)

Herpes simplex virus

1 Viral characteristics:
  (a) DNA virus, usually type I, occasionally type II; intracellular infection
  (b) diagnosis: electron micrograph of affected cells, aspirate from blisters, viral culture, monoclonal antibody staining, serial serum antibody titres
  (c) primary infection; self limiting periocular vesicles and crusting, follicular and papillary blepharoconjunctivitis

after

after 1° infect retrograde to ganglia — latent —> reactivate — anterograde to the skin / eye

    (d) recurrent infection caused by reactivation of dormant virus in trigeminal ganglion or cornea; causes superficial and stromal keratitis

    (e) 5 year recurrence rate: 25% after first episode, 50% after subsequent episodes

2 Dendritic ulcer:
    (a) epithelial disease
    (b) early coarse punctate or stellate pattern
    (c) later characteristic branching pattern
    (d) ulcer bed stains with fluorescein, margin with rose Bengal
    (e) corneal sensitivity diminished
    (f) anterior stromal infiltrates after a few days
    (g) heals in 1–2 weeks, with scarring *if this happens*

3 Geographic ulcer
    (a) enlarged superficial amoeboid ulcer
    (b) usually in association with topical steroid treatment (without antiviral agents)
    (c) all have stromal involvement

4 Trophic keratitis:
    (a) metaherpetic disease, not caused by active virus
    (b) due to persistent defect in epithelial basement membrane
    (c) similar to recurrent corneal erosions

5 Stromal infiltrative keratitis: *(Keratouveitis)*
    (a) active viral invasion and stromal destruction
    (b) cheesy, necrotic, stromal appearance
    (c) associated anterior uveitis and keratic precipitates (KPs)
    (d) may ulcerate
    (e) thinning and vascularised scarring results

6 Disciform keratitis:
    (a) type IV hypersensitivity reaction
    (b) typical central, epithelial, and stromal oedema
    (c) folds in Descemet's membrane
    (d) mild to moderate anterior uveitis, with KPs
    (e) may have surrounding ring of cellular infiltrate and antibody–antigen reaction (Wessely ring)
    (f) reduced corneal sensation
    (g) nebular scarring may result

7 Complications:
    (a) uveitis *granulomatous —> PS + iris patch atrophy*
    (b) glaucoma
    (c) episcleritis
    (d) scleritis
    (e) secondary bacterial infections
    (f) perforation

systemic disseminated HSV inf —> encephitis
— full thickness bilat. Retinal oedematous retn. whitening vasculitis + occlusion

8 Management:
    (a) treat superficial lesions with topical antiviral agents (acyclovir, trifluorothymidine, idoxuridine, vidarabine) and/or débridement
    (b) disciform keratitis requires topical steroid and antiviral agents
    (c) geographic ulcers require topical antivirals usually in combination with topical steroids

Cong — type II at birth
— keratitis
— iridocyclitis
— Cataract
— optic atrophy ± retinitis

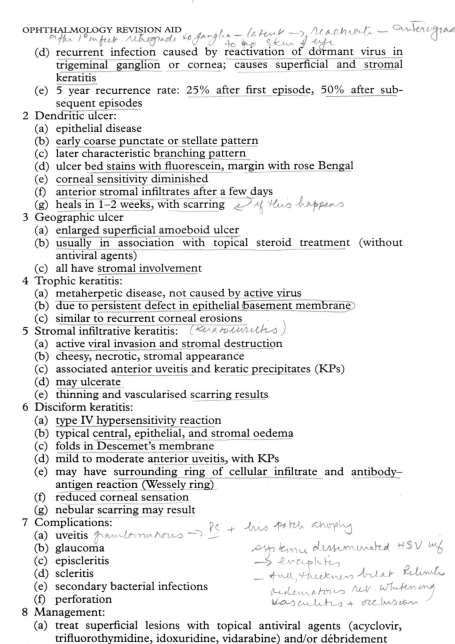

(d) trophic keratitis requires lubricant ointments and padding; may need a bandage contact lens

(e) topical cycloplegics to relieve ciliary and sphincter spasm, and prevent synechiae

Herpes zoster keratitis

1 Viral characteristics:
   (a) varicella-zoster (DNA) virus
   (b) previous systemic infection (chickenpox) usually between ages 3 and 10 years (primary)
   (c) virus lies dormant in sensory nerve root ganglion
   (d) affects older age group and immunosuppressed; M = F
   (e) diagnose with electron micrography, viral culture, monoclonal antibody staining, serial serum antibody titres
   (f) herpes zoster ophthalmicus accounts for 7% of all shingles

2 General features:
   (a) painful, red, vesicular rash, progressing to crusting, and resolution often with scarring
   (b) general malaise, lethargy, depression
   (c) occasional dehydration
   (d) postherpetic neuralgia (50% of these >70 years; rare <60 years)

3 Ocular features:
   (a) occur in 50%; ocular involvement more common if nasociliary branch of Va affected
   (b) mucopurulent conjunctivitis
   (c) episcleritis
   (d) scleritis
   (e) keratitis:
       (i) peripheral microdendrites
       (ii) punctate epithelial erosions
       (iii) filamentary keratitis
       (iv) nummular keratitis
       (v) disciform keratitis
       (vi) neurotrophic keratitis
       (vii) mucous plaque keratitis
   (f) uveitis in 50% with segmental iris atrophy
   (g) glaucoma
   (h) ophthalmoplegia
   (i) lid scarring with resultant ptosis, trichiasis, ectropion, entropion
   (j) may get relapsing keratouveitis
   (k) optic neuritis

4 Neurological features:
   (a) cranial nerve palsies
   (b) optic neuritis
   (c) encephalitis
   (d) contralateral hemiplegia (rare)

5 Management:
   (a) bedrest, prevention of dehydration, analgesia, and general supportive measures

(b) systemic antiviral agents in acute stage (acyclovir or newer agents, e.g. valaciclovir/famciclovir), especially if patient immuno-compromised
(c) topical antiviral agents in vesicular stage, e.g. acyclovir cream to skin, ointment to eye (if involved) ? ?
(d) skin emollients in crusting stage and treat any secondary infections
(e) topical steroids if keratitis causing scarring or severe uveitis (withdraw slowly as steroid dependency results)
(f) topical cycloplegics to relieve ciliary and sphincter spasm, and prevent synechiae

Causes of disciform keratitis

1 Herpes simplex
2 Herpes zoster
3 Trauma
4 Vaccinia (cowpox)
5 Syphilis

Fungal and yeast infections

1 Rare
2 Usually *Aspergillus*, *Fusarium*, or *Candida* spp.
3 In immunocompromised hosts/with topical steroids/trauma with organic contamination
4 Suspect in suppurative/necrotic keratitis
5 Identify with Giemsa staining
6 Culture with Sabouraud's agar and brain–heart infusion medium
7 Treat fungi with topical 5% natamycin
8 Treat yeasts with topical and oral flucytosine

Protozoan/worm/spirochaete infections

1 Acanthamoebae:
   (a) rare, but increasing number of cases in recent years
   (b) predisposing causes:
       (i) soft contact lenses
       (ii) swimming in freshwater lakes and "hot tubs"
   (c) persistent keratitis resistant to treatment with antibiotics and steroids; epithelial breakdown; ring infiltrate with prominent corneal nerves caused by radial perineuritis; hypopyon, hyphaema, and secondary glaucoma; severe pain and chemosis out of propor-tion with keratitis
   (d) diagnosis: deep corneal scraping or histology of recipient corneal button; culture on *Escherichia coli* or *Enterobacter aerogenes* enriched non-nutrient agar plates; staining including Giemsa, PAS, calco-fluor white, and fluorescent antibody
   (e) treatment:
       (i) dibromopropamidine ointment
       (ii) propamidine drops
       (iii) neomycin drops + PHMB (polyhexamethylbiguanide)

    (iv) keratoplasty

    (v) antibiotics for any secondary infection

    (vi) steroids

    (vii) treatment of any associated glaucoma

2 Interstitial keratitis:
  (a) most common cause is congenital syphilis
  (b) acute stromal keratitis with oedema and vascularisation ("salmon patch keratitis")
  (c) accompanying granulomatous uveitis
  (d) resolves to leave a stromal nebula with characteristic "ghost vessels"
  (e) other causes: tuberculosis, mumps, varicella, brucellosis, malaria, onchocerciasis, trypanosomiasis, herpes simplex

MECHANICAL TRAUMA

1 Scarring only if Bowman's or deeper layers are involved
2 Recurrent erosions can occur following abrasions
3 Disciform keratitis with blunt trauma

ALKALI INJURIES

1 Alkalis in decreasing order of tissue penetrability and potential damage:
  (a) ammonium hydroxide
  (b) sodium hydroxide
  (c) potassium hydroxide
  (d) calcium hydroxide
  (e) magnesium hydroxide
2 Acute features (up to 1 week):
  (a) partial or total conjunctival and epithelial loss
  (b) corneal clouding and oedema
  (c) ischaemia from thrombosis of conjunctival, episcleral (and scleral) vessels
  (d) if severe: fibrinous uveitis, acute glaucoma or hypotony, thrombosis of iris vessels, cataract
  (e) damage varies with alkali type, pH, quantity, area and duration of exposure
  (f) caused by lipid saponification and proteolysis
3 Grading the injury:
  (a) grade I: corneal epithelial damage, no ischaemia, good prognosis (full recovery)
  (b) grade II: cornea hazy but iris details seen; ischaemia of $<\frac{1}{3}$ at the limbus; good prognosis (some scarring)
  (c) grade III: total loss of corneal epithelium; stromal haze obscures iris details; ischaemia of $\frac{1}{3}$ to $\frac{1}{2}$ at the limbus, guarded prognosis (vision impaired, perforation rare)
  (d) grade IV: cornea opaque obscuring view of iris and pupil; ischaemia of more than $\frac{1}{2}$ at the limbus; poor prognosis (perforation common)

4 Early reparative phase (1–3 weeks):
   (a) regeneration of corneal/conjunctival epithelium (unless grade IV)
   (b) resolution of uveitis (unless grade III or IV)
   (c) corneal neovascularisation commences (in grades II, III, IV)
   (d) progressive/recurrent corneal ulceration (grades III and IV)
5 Late reparative phase (after 3 weeks) (grades II, III, IV injuries only):
   (a) corneal neovascularisation and scarring
   (b) corneal ulceration persists or progresses to perforation
   (c) conjunctival and episcleral scarring, and keratinisation
   (d) symblepharon, entropion, trichiasis
   (e) tear film abnormalities
   (f) neurotrophic keratitis
6 Immediate treatment:
   (a) copious irrigation with water, physiological saline, or buffered solutions
   (b) monitor pH
   (c) removal of solid foreign material and necrotic tissue (including double eversion of lids to remove subtarsal foreign material)
7 Further management of grade I/II burns:
   (a) topical antibiotics, cycloplegics
   (b) 10% ascorbate drops (aid collagen synthesis, scavenger for damaging superoxide radicals)
   (c) daily forniceal rodding (or scleral lenses) to prevent symblepharon
   (d) topical steroids (with caution) for first 10 days
   (e) subconjunctival injection of heparinised blood
8 Further management of grade III/IV burns:
   (a) as for grade I/II but avoid topical steroids
   (b) topical collagenase inhibitors (cysteine or disodium EDTA)
   (c) early conjunctival and/or corneal grafting

ACID INJURIES

1 Acids in decreasing order of potential ocular damage:
   (a) hydrofluoric acid
      sulphuric acid
      sulphurous acid
      chromic acid
   (b) hydrochloric acid
      nitric acid
   (c) acetic acid
2 Acid injuries are similar to alkali injuries but less severe as a result of self limiting coagulation of surface epithelium
3 Management is similar to that for alkali injuries

RADIATION INJURIES

1 Thermal burns are similar to acid burns
2 Ultraviolet radiation:
   (a) causes a punctate epithelial keratitis

(b) arises 8–12 hours following exposure ("arc eye", "welder's flash", and "snow blindness")
(c) resolves completely
3 Ionising radiation:
   (a) initial superficial keratitis
   (b) later stromal disruption as a result of keratocyte damage
   (c) corneal drying secondary to keratinisation of conjunctiva
   (d) loss of goblet cells from conjunctiva

PERIPHERAL CORNEAL ULCERATION

1 Marginal ulcer:
   (a) initial subepithelial infiltrate with peripheral clear zone
   (b) progresses to small shallow ulcer
   (c) hypersensitivity reaction to staphylococcal exotoxins
   (d) resolves spontaneously
   (e) topical steroids help
   (f) treat any underlying blepharitis
2 Mooren's ulcer:
   (a) rare, unknown aetiology
   (b) chronic peripheral thinning or melt
   (c) painful
   (d) blurring caused by irregular astigmatism
   (e) often superior; spreading circumferentially
   (f) may perforate
   (g) frequently unresponsive to treatment
   (h) exclude a predisposing scleritis
3 Terrien's marginal degeneration:
   (a) bilateral
   (b) peripheral corneal thinning
   (c) painless
   (d) often men over 40
   (e) early yellowish stromal opacities in upper cornea
   (f) slowly progresses to non-staining gutter
   (g) vision may be impaired as a result of astigmatism
   (h) may perforate or need tectonic graft

Systemic disorders associated with peripheral corneal ulceration

1 Rheumatoid arthritis (seropositive)
2 Systemic lupus erythematosus
3 Polyarteritis nodosa
4 Scleroderma
5 Wegener's granulomatosis
6 Giant cell arteritis
7 Relapsing polychondritis
8 Acute leukaemia
9 Gold toxicity
10 Bacillary dysentery

11 Syphilis
12 Rosacea

CORNEAL DEPOSITS

1 Wilson's disease:
  (a) Kayser–Fleischer ring (copper in Descemet's membrane)
  (b) "sunflower cataract"
2 Mucopolysaccharidoses:
  (a) only Hurler's, Scheie's, Morquio's, Maroteaux–Lamy
  (b) stromal deposition
3 Verticillata:
  (a) vortex pattern of epithelial deposition
  (b) in Fabry's disease
  (c) in systemic drug therapy:
      (i) chloroquine
      (ii) amiodarone
      (iii) chlorpromazine
      (iv) indomethacin
4 Crystalline deposits in: *stromal (ant)*
  (a) cystinosis
  (b) oxalosis
  (c) gout
  (d) gold therapy
  (e) argyrosis
  (f) multiple myeloma
  (g) Waldenström's macroglobulinaemia
  (h) lymphoma
  (i) Schnyder's central crystalline keratopathy *Cholesterol within keratocytes*
5 Iron deposition:
  (a) epithelial:
      (i) keratoconus (Fleischer's ring)
      (ii) pterygium (Stocker's line)
      (iii) filtering bleb (Ferry's line)
      (iv) old age (Hudson–Stahli line)
      (v) following excimer laser PRK
  (b) stromal:
      (i) siderosis
      (ii) black ball hyphaema

CORNEAL TOXICITY

1 Preservatives:
  (a) whorled pattern of punctate epithelial erosions
  (b) superior pannus and erosions (with thiomersal)
2 Antiviral agents:
  (a) inhibit epithelial regeneration
  (b) cause punctate epitheliopathy
  (c) include idoxuridine, acyclovir, vidarabine, trifluorothymidine

ROSACEA KERATITIS

1 Peripheral vascularisation, typically in the 4 and 8 o'clock positions
2 Corneal thinning
3 Punctate epithelial erosions in lower $\frac{2}{3}$
4 Recurrent epithelial erosions in upper cornea
5 Map/dot subepithelial opacities
6 Ultimately neovascularisation and scarring

VERNAL KERATOPATHY

1 Punctate epithelial erosions in upper cornea
2 Vernal ulcer; painless, circumscribed, oval ulcer in upper cornea, often with a plaque of exudate and mucus in the base
3 Subepithelial "ring" scar; caused by healed ulcer
4 Pseudogerontotoxon
5 Treat with:
   (a) topical steroids
   (b) sodium cromoglycate drops
   (c) acetylcysteine drops
   (d) débridement of ulcer base
   (e) oral antihistamines

EXPOSURE KERATOPATHY

1 Corneal drying
2 Punctate epithelial erosions
3 Can progress to ulceration with infection
4 Causes:
   (a) proptosis
   (b) nerve VII palsy
   (c) severe ectropion
   (d) coma
   (e) lid trauma
   (f) ptosis over-correction

NEUROTROPHIC KERATOPATHY

1 Anaesthetic cornea
2 Precise pathological process is unclear
3 Punctate epithelial erosions (especially interpalpebral)
4 Can progress to ulceration
5 Causes:
   (a) herpes zoster ophthalmicus
   (b) herpes simplex
   (c) trigeminal nerve damage
   (d) diabetes mellitus
   (e) leprosy
   (f) familial dysautonomia

  (g) anhidrotic ectodermal dysplasia
  (h) congenital insensitivity to pain

KERATOMALACIA

1 Corneal melt with xerosis
2 Due to vitamin A deficiency
3 Conjunctival keratinisation and drying
4 Increased incidence of infection
5 Ulceration and perforation
6 Other causes:
  (a) scleroderma
  (b) Wegener's granulomatosis
  (c) cytomegalovirus
  (d) rheumatoid arthritis

EPISCLERITIS

1 Features:
  (a) inflammation of episclera and overlying conjunctiva; blanches with phenylephrine drops
  (b) nodular or diffuse
  (c) benign and self limiting
  (d) more common in young adults; M = F
  (e) mild ache, tenderness, burning
  (f) occasionally associated with systemic disease, e.g. herpes zoster ophthalmicus, rheumatoid arthritis, and hyperuricaemia
2 Treatment:
  (a) topical steroids and/or oxyphenbutazone
  (b) systemic non-steroidal anti-inflammatory drugs (NSAIDs)
  (c) none (condition self limiting)

SCLERITIS

1 Less common but more serious than episcleritis
2 Often very painful, but can very occasionally be painless
3 Pain may be worse at night
4 Especially affecting older women.

Anterior scleritis

1 Diffuse non-necrotising:
  (a) segmented or widespread inflammation of anterior sclera
  (b) oedema with distortion of deep vascular plexus
  (c) treat with oral NSAIDs, e.g. flurbiprofen
2 Nodular non-necrotising:
  (a) focal scleral inflammation and oedema
  (b) nodule is immobile
  (c) treat with oral non-steroidal anti-inflammatory drugs, e.g. indomethacin

3 Necrotising, without inflammation:
  (a) scleromalacia perforans
  (b) in seropositive rheumatoid arthritis
  (c) painless scleral thinning with marked ischaemia
  (d) seldom perforate
  (e) treatment is difficult
4 Necrotising, with inflammation:
  (a) progressive, red, and painful
  (b) vascular sludging and occlusion; scleral ischaemia and non-perfusion
  (c) focal or diffuse
  (d) associated anterior uveitis
  (e) scleral thinning
  (f) 25% five year mortality from associated disease
  (g) severe complications, e.g. sclerosing keratitis, peripheral corneal melts, cataract, glaucoma
  (h) treat with high dose systemic steroids, sometimes in combination with immunosuppressive drugs, e.g. azathioprine, cyclophosphamide, cyclosporin
  (i) subconjunctival steroids contraindicated

Posterior scleritis

1 Features:
  (a) thickened and inflamed posterior sclera
  (b) anterior segment may be unaffected
  (c) easily missed
  (d) may have ocular pain or may be painless
  (e) exudative retinal detachment
  (f) thickened posterior sclera (diffuse or focal)
  (g) choroidal folds
  (h) posterior vitritis, and disc and macular oedema
  (i) uveal effusion syndrome
  (j) proptosis
  (k) ocular myositis with ophthalmoplegia
  (l) usually no associated systemic disorder
2 Investigations: CT scan or ultrasonic B scan may help diagnosis because of thickened sclera
3 Treatment: high dose systemic steroids or immunosuppressive drugs

Systemic diseases associated with scleritis

1 Herpes zoster ophthalmicus
2 Rheumatoid arthritis
3 Systemic lupus erythematosus
4 Polyarteritis nodosa
5 Wegener's granulomatosis
6 Relapsing polychondritis
7 Dermatomyositis
8 Sarcoidosis

9 Behçet's syndrome
10 Ankylosing spondylitis
11 Crohn's disease
12 Ulcerative colitis
13 Gout

6
UVEITIS AND ENDOPHTHALMITIS

UVEITIS

Nomenclature

Uveitis: inflammation of the uveal tract

Anterior uveitis: mainly iris (iritis) and ciliary body (cyclitis) inflammation, e.g. in ankylosing spondylitis

Intermediate uveitis and pars planitis

Posterior uveitis: mainly choroidal inflammation (choroiditis), e.g. in tuberculosis

Panuveitis: inflammation of all parts of the uveal tract, e.g. sympathetic ophthalmia

Symptoms

1 Photophobia
2 Pain (deep ocular pain) worsened by accommodation
3 Reflex lacrimation
4 Reduced visual acuity
5 "Floaters"

Anterior segment signs of uveitis

[handwritten: inflam in the A/c to require Rx for ≥ 3/12]

1 Ciliary injection (circumcorneal flush from branches of anterior ciliary arteries and ciliary efferent veins from ciliary venous plexus)
2 Conjunctival and episcleral injection (severe anterior uveitis)
3 Small pupils (iris sphincter spasm)
4 Flare in anterior chamber (turbid aqueous humour)
5 Inflammatory cells in anterior chamber
6 Inflammatory cells on endothelium ("keratic precipitates" which are described as "mutton fat" if large with waxy or fatty appearance)
7 Iris nodules:
   (a) Koeppe's (pupil margin)
   (b) Busacca's (anterior iris stroma)
8 Hypopyon
9 Dilated iris vessels, occasionally new vessels (rubeosis)

*[handwritten: of cases 50% HLA B27 (normal pop 8%)
B27+ve – sever reaction
– extensive PS
Dm type II – hypopyon.]*

75

10 Synechiae:
    (a) posterior (iris adhesions to lens): seclusio pupillae (complete 360° adhesion) may lead to obstruction of aqueous flow through pupil, resulting in "iris bombé" and angle closure glaucoma
    (b) anterior (iris adhesions to drainage angle and cornea)
11 Iris atrophy ⎫
12 Band keratopathy ⎬ longstanding uveitis
13 Secondary cataract ⎭

Posterior segment signs of uveitis

1 Vitreous cells
2 Vitreous membranes and opacities
3 Inflammatory exudates, e.g. peripheral retinal "snowbanking"
4 Vasculitis: opacification around vessels e.g. periphlebitis and sheathing:
    (a) Cotton wool spots
    (b) Exudates
5 Retinitis: colour depends on stage of lesion, white in acute stage, greyish later on
6 Retinal detachment: serous or rhegmatogenous
7 Pigmentary changes: hypo- and hyperpigmentation secondary to inflammation in retinal pigment epithelium
8 Choroiditis:
    (a) focal ⎫ fluorescein angiography may
    (b) multifocal ⎬ occasionally be helpful in
    (c) diffuse ⎭ distinguishing
9 Choroidal detachment
10 Neovascularisation (may be ischaemic or inflammatory, retinal, or subretinal)
11 Macular oedema
12 Optic disc swelling and atrophy

Classification

1 Idiopathic (largest group)
2 Associated with systemic disease:
    (a) ankylosing spondylitis
    (b) Reiter's syndrome
    (c) psoriatic arthritis
    (d) inflammatory bowel disease
    (e) juvenile chronic arthritis
    (f) sarcoidosis
    (g) Behçet's syndrome
    (h) multiple sclerosis
3 Infectious causes:
    (a) bacterial:
        (i) tuberculosis
        (ii) syphilis
        (iii) gonorrhoea
        (iv) leprosy

    (b) viral:
- (i) herpes simplex
- (ii) herpes zoster
- (iii) HIV
- (iv) measles

    (c) fungal:
- (i) presumed ocular histoplasmosis syndrome
- (ii) coccidioidomycosis
- (iii) candidiasis

    (d) infestations:
- (i) toxoplasmosis
- (ii) toxocariasis
- (iii) onchocerciasis

4 Specific uveitis entities:
- (a) Fuchs' heterochromic cyclitis
- (b) Vogt–Koyanagi–Harada syndrome
- (c) sympathetic ophthalmia
- (d) birdshot retinochoroidopathy
- (e) acute multifocal placoid pigment epitheliopathy (AMPPE)
- (f) serpiginous choroidopathy
- (g) acute retinal necrosis
- (h) sarcoidosis

5 Lens induced:
- (a) phakoanaphylactic uveitis

6 Masquerade syndromes:
- (a) non-Hodgkin's lymphoma
- (b) melanoma
- (c) retinoblastoma *(in children – occ in A/c)*

General signs and symptoms

1 Joint problems:
- (a) ankylosing spondylitis
- (b) juvenile chronic arthritis
- (c) Reiter's syndrome
- (d) inflammatory bowel disease
- (e) Behçet's syndrome
- (f) Whipple's disease
- (g) sarcoidosis
- (h) leprosy
- (i) metastatic gonococcal disease

2 Diarrhoea:
- (a) inflammatory bowel disease
- (b) Whipple's disease

3 Influenza-like illness:
- (a) toxoplasmosis
- (b) leptospirosis
- (c) histoplasmosis

4 Jaundice:
- (a) leptospirosis

77

    (b) inflammatory bowel disease
5 Liver enlargement:
    (a) toxocariasis
    (b) cytomegalovirus
    (c) toxoplasmosis
6 Central nervous system involvement:
    (a) TB meningitis
    (b) Vogt–Koyanagi–Harada syndrome
    (c) congenital toxoplasmosis
    (d) congenital cytomegalovirus
    (e) Behçet's disease
    (f) non-Hodgkin's lymphoma
    (g) tertiary syphilis
    (h) multiple sclerosis
7 Skin rash:
    (a) secondary syphilis
    (b) sarcoidosis
    (c) Behçet's disease
    (d) psoriasis
    (e) Reiter's syndrome
    (f) Vogt–Koyanagi–Harada syndrome
    (g) histoplasmosis
    (h) herpes simplex
    (i) herpes zoster
8 Erythema nodosum:
    (a) sarcoidosis
    (b) tuberculosis
    (c) inflammatory bowel disease
    (d) histoplasmosis
    (e) AMPPE
    (f) Behçet's disease
9 Chest symptoms:
    (a) tuberculosis
    (b) sarcoidosis
10 Urinary disorders:
    (a) Reiter's syndrome
    (b) metastatic gonococcal disease
    (c) Behçet's syndrome
11 Mouth ulcers:
    (a) Behçet's syndrome
    (b) Reiter's syndrome
    (c) herpes simplex
    (d) inflammatory bowel disease

Conditions resembling anterior uveitis *masquarading syndrom*

1 Microhyphaema
2 Pigment in the anterior chamber (often after mydriasis)
3 Malignant lymphomas or leukaemia or histiocytic lymphoma
4 Retinoblastoma

5 Pseudoexfoliation of the lens capsule
6 Ghost cell glaucoma

Grading of uveitis

Table 6.1   Cells

Grade	Cells per field
0	0
+	1–10
+ +	11–20
+ + +	21–50
+ + + +	> 50

Slitlamp beam width = 1 mm; length = 3 mm. Cells counted within this field.

Table 6.2   Flare

Grading of flare	Description
0	Complete absence
+	Faint = barely detectable
+ +	Moderate = iris and lens details clear
+ + +	Marked = iris and lens details hazy
+ + + +	Intense = fibrinous aqueous

To grade flare: same setting on slitlamp as for counting cells.

Table 6.3   Vitritis

Grade	Description
0	Clear vitreous
+	Diffuse scattered opacities, fundal view unimpaired
+ +	Moderate scattered opacities, fundal detail somewhat obscured
+ + +	Many opacities, marked blurring of fundal details
+ + + +	Dense opacities, no fundus views

SYSTEMIC DISORDERS ASSOCIATED WITH UVEITIS

Ankylosing spondylitis
Affects young men; 90% HLA-B27 positive.
1 General features:
    (a) arthritis: sacroiliac joints and peripheral joints
    (b) heart: aortic incompetence
    (c) colitis (10%)
    (d) lungs: apical fibrosis and restricted chest expansion, kyphoscoliosis
2 Ocular features:
    (a) acute anterior uveitis; recurrent attacks in 40%
    (b) episcleritis

Reiter's syndrome

Triad of conjunctivitis, urethritis, and arthritis; 70% patients HLA-B27 positive, M >> F.

1 General features:
  (a) urethritis (non-specific)
  (b) may follow dysentery
  (c) arthritis: knees, sacroiliac joints, ankles
  (d) plantar fasciitis and Achilles tendinitis
  (e) keratoderma blenorrhagica on feet and hands
  (f) circinate balanitis
  (g) painless mouth ulcers
2 Ocular features:
  (a) mucopurulent conjunctivitis
  (b) keratitis with anterior stromal infiltrates
  (c) acute anterior uveitis (30%)

Psoriatic arthritis   *remember no Psoriasis but psoriatic arthritis*

Increased incidence in patients with HLA-B17 and HLA-B27.

1 General features:
  (a) arthritis usually affecting hands, feet, and sacroiliac joints; occurs in 5% of patients with psoriasis
  (b) psoriatic skin and nail changes
2 Ocular features:
  (a) conjunctivitis
  (b) acute anterior uveitis
  (c) dry eyes

Inflammatory bowel disease (Crohn's disease, ulcerative colitis)

1 General features:
  (a) arthritis
  (b) erythema nodosum
  (c) hepatitis
  (d) sclerosing cholangitis
  (e) pyoderma gangrenosum
2 Ocular features:
  (a) conjunctivitis
  (b) keratoconjunctivitis sicca
  (c) keratoconjunctivitis
  (d) episcleritis and scleritis
  (e) anterior uveitis
  (f) retinal oedema
  (g) orbital cellulitis
  (h) optic neuritis

Juvenile chronic arthritis (JCA)

Seronegative arthritis in patients ≤16 years of age.

1 General features:
  (a) arthritis: pauciarticular if less than 5 joints affected

Systemic

polyarticular — > 5 joints

pauciarticular — early ↓10, ♀, ANA +ve, long course Rh −ve; late ↑10 − ♂, ANA −ve, Rh −ve, acute, recu...

(b) fever
(c) lymphadenopathy ⎫ 30% of children with JCA
(d) maculopapular (rash) ⎬ present with these systemic
(e) hepatosplenomegaly ⎪ features
(f) myocarditis ⎭
2 Ocular features:
  (a) chronic anterior uveitis (70% bilateral); increased risk in: + *PS*
    ✗ (i) pauciarticular arthritis
    ✗ (ii) girl with anti-nuclear antibodies✗
  (b) secondary glaucoma (20%) – *genitourny, systemi CME*
  (c) cataract (40%) *linsectomy + Vitrectomy .no IOL, no PC,*
  (d) secondary band keratopathy (40%) *DETA.*

Causes of anterior uveitis in childhood

1 Juvenile chronic arthritis ⎫ these account for most cases
2 Juvenile ankylosing spondylitis ⎬
3 Psoriatic arthritis
4 Reiter's syndrome
5 Behçet's syndrome
6 Vogt–Koyanagi–Harada syndrome
7 Sarcoidosis
8 Idiopathic iridocyclitis
9 Heterochromic cyclitis
10 Pars planitis

Sarcoidosis

A multisystem granulomatous disease of unknown aetiology; usually affects young adults; F > M.
1 Presentations:
  (a) Löfgren's syndrome:
    (i) acute onset
    (ii) hilar lymphadenopathy
    (iii) erythema nodosum
    (iv) anterior uveitis
    (v) arthralgia
  (b) Mikulicz's syndrome:
    (i) lacrimal and parotid gland swelling
    (ii) sicca syndrome
    (iii) causes:
      • sarcoidosis
      • tuberculosis
      • lymphoma
      • leukaemia
  (c) Heerfordt's syndrome:
    (i) parotid gland enlargement
    (ii) fever
    (iii) anterior uveitis
    (iv) facial nerve palsy

2 General features:
  (a) lungs:
      (i) hilar lymphadenopathy
      (ii) diffuse fibrosis
  (b) skin:
      (i) lupus pernio
      (ii) erythema nodosum
  (c) bones and joints:
      (i) arthralgia
      (ii) cystic bony lesions in phalanges
  (d) visceral organs: hepatosplenomegaly
  (e) nervous system: peripheral neuropathy and cranial nerve lesions
  (f) endocrine: diabetes insipidus
3 Ocular features:
  (a) eyelids may be involved by purple sarcoid indurating rash (lupus pernio)
  (b) band keratopathy
  (c) lacrimal gland infiltration with enlargement
  (d) conjunctival follicles
  (e) episcleritis and scleritis with nodules
  (f) anterior uveitis:
      (i) acute—particularly in Löfgren's syndrome
      (ii) chronic—classically of granulomatous type with mutton fat keratic precipitates
  (g) secondary cataracts and glaucoma
  (h) vitritis (classic sign)
  (i) choroiditis with yellow or white nodules
  (j) retinal periphlebitis with candle wax retinal exudates
  (k) retinal neovascularisation
  (l) pars planitis
  (m) choroidal granulomata
  (n) optic nerve granuloma
  (o) disc oedema

Behçet's disease

Triad of oral ulceration, genital ulceration, and inflammatory eye lesions; M>F; more common in Japan and the Mediterranean; increased prevalence of HLA-B5. / B5/
1 General features:
  (a) oral ulceration
  (b) genital ulceration
  (c) skin lesions including erythema nodosum
  (d) arthritis
  (e) thrombophlebitis (associated with Vena Cava thrombosis)
  (f) large vessel occlusion.
  (g) gastrointestinal: pain, diarrhoea, constipation, and ulceration
  (h) meningoencephalitis
2 Ocular features:
  (a) anterior uveitis (sometimes with hypopyon) hypopyon may resolve spontaneously.

Characteristic sign ⌐ anter, periphery
                                              └ hypopyon
                                              └ niemen BRVO + Ischemia

(b) conjunctivitis
(c) keratitis
(d) episcleritis
(e) retinal vasculitis with retinal infarction
(f) branch vein occlusion *ischemi/recurrent.*
(g) neovascularisation with vitreous haemorrhage *-2° rubeotic glaucoma + phthisc*
(h) retinal and macular oedema
(i) retinal exudates in the outer retinal layers *Characteristic - peripheral retina larger than CWS.*

Choroid is not involved

INFECTIONS

Tuberculosis

Disease caused by infection with *Mycobacterium tuberculosis*.
1 Ocular features:
  (a) lupus vulgaris on the eyelids
  (b) ectropion from scarring around sinuses from discharging orbital lesions
  (c) conjunctiva:
      (i) phlyctenular conjunctivitis.
      (ii) primary conjunctival tuberculosis
  (d) keratitis
  (e) scleritis
  (f) lacrimal gland involvement
  (g) orbital periostitis
  (h) granulomatous panuveitis (ciliary body and iris nodules)
  (i) secondary glaucoma and cataract
  (j) choroidoretinal plaque or nodule (tuberculoma)
  (k) non-rhegmatogenous retinal detachment *exudative/serous*
  (l) cranial nerve palsies (basal meningitis)

Acquired syphilis

Disease caused by infection with *Treponema pallidum*.
1 Stages:
  (a) primary: characterised by ulcerating painless lesion (chancre)
  (b) secondary:
      (i) maculopapular rash
      (ii) lymphadenopathy
      (iii) fever
      (iv) malaise
      (v) condylomata lata
      (vi) hepatitis
      (vii) periostitis *-bone + dental abnormalities* [*Hutchinson teeth. Sabre tibia Saddle nose deformities*]
  (c) tertiary: local tissue destruction by chronic inflammation in any part of the body (gumma):
      (i) CNS:
        • meningoencephalitis
        • general paralysis of the insane
        • tabes dorsalis
      (ii) CVS:

83

Serologiueas:
- direct (previous + current — (FTA-Abs)
  activity — MHA-TP)
- indirect - disease activity — VDRL
  RPR

Rx — Systemic penicillin
  + Probenecid
  topical steroid + mydriatic

- aortic aneurysm
- aortic incompetence

2 Ocular features:
  (a) hyperaemic changes in superficial vascular loops of the iris (transient roseolae)
  (b) iris papules and gummas (yellow–red nodules)
  (c) panuveitis resistant to treatment.
  (d) choroidoretinitis (localised or diffuse); may mimic retinitis pigmentosa
  (e) optic neuritis or optic atrophy
  (f) Argyll Robertson pupils
  (g) madarosis: loss of eyebrows and eyelashes

Congenital syphilis

1 General features:
  (a) death *in utero* or perinatal
  (b) inflammation of internal organs
  (c) dental abnormalities (Hutchinson's teeth)
  (d) facial deformities including "saddle" nose
  (e) CNS disease; nerve deafness
2 Ocular features:
  (a) interstitial keratitis (keratouveitis): 5–25 years of age; new vessels create "salmon patch" in cornea; vessels then atrophy ("ghost" vessels) although corneal scar remains
  (b) anterior uveitis in association with keratitis
  (c) dislocated lens — Cataract. → glaucoma.
  (d) Argyll Robertson pupils
  (e) optic atrophy
  (f) choroidoretinitis:
      (i) diffuse ("salt and pepper" fundus)
      (ii) focal

Leprosy

Chronic granulomatous infection caused by *Mycobacterium leprae*. A spectrum of disease depending on cellular immunity to infecting organism, from tuberculous leprosy (high immunity) to lepromatous leprosy (low immunity).
1 Ocular features:
  (a) lids: lagophthalmos, madarosis, blepharochalasis, nodules, trichiasis, ectropion and entropion, and reduced blinking
  (b) lacrimal: acute and chronic dacryocystitis
  (c) cornea: anaesthesia, exposure keratopathy, band keratopathy, corneal leproma, interstitial keratitis, (thickened) corneal nerves, and superficial stromal keratitis
  (d) sclera: episcleritis, scleritis, staphyloma, and nodules
  (e) iris: miosis, acute and chronic iritis, leading to synechiae, seclusio pupillae, cataract, glaucoma, iris atrophy, iris pearls, and leproma
  (f) ciliary: hypotonia, phthisis, and loss of accommodation — microleproma small white
  (g) fundus: peripheral choroidal lesions, retinal vasculitis
  very suggestive of leprosy.

Sympathetic neuropathy

84 generally - skin lesions
  - sensory loss
  - enlarged peripheral nerves.
Rx Dapsone + Rifampicin topical steroid + mydriasis

Cytomegalovirus disease (in immunosuppressed host)

Ocular features:
  (a) mild anterior uveitis may be present
  (b) retinal ischaemia and necrosis
  (c) multiple haemorrhages
  (d) vascular sheathing; occlusion
  (e) optic nerve involvement, oedema, and suboptic atrophy
  (f) widespread retinitis and haemorrhages

Measles (rubeola)—myxovirus

Ocular features:
  (a) keratoconjunctivitis: blinding disease in malnourished patients with vitamin A deficiency
  (b) retinal oedema
  (c) vascular attenuation
  (d) macular star

Subacute sclerosing panencephalitis (SSPE)

1 General features:
  (a) personality or behavioural changes
  (b) dementia
  (c) seizures
  (d) myoclonus
2 Ocular features (50%):
  (a) macular or paramacular choroidoretinitis
  (b) pigmentary changes with bone corpuscle configuration
  (c) papilloedema
  (d) optic atrophy
  (e) nystagmus
  (f) cortical blindness

Candidiasis

1 Occurs in compromised host:
  (a) immunosuppressants, steroids, HIV infection
  (b) drug addicts using intravenous injections
  (c) long term indwelling catheters
2 Ocular features:
  (a) anterior uveitis
  (b) retinal haemorrhage and perivascular sheathing
  (c) chorioretinitis starts with white fluffy lesions ("puff-balls"); these lesions may be joined by opaque vitreous strands giving rise to the "string-of-pearls" sign; proceeds to:
  (d) vitreous abscess formation

Presumed ocular histoplasmosis syndrome (POHS)

Infection caused by fungus *Histoplasma capsulatum*. Endemic in certain river valleys between 45° north and 45° south. POHS seen in patients with

85

no clinical or no serological evidence of histoplasma infection, hence "presumed" label. Higher prevalence of HLA-B7.

1 Ocular features:
   (a) multifocal atrophic choroidal lesions *punched out when atrophic*
   (b) peripapillary atrophy
   (c) disciform maculopathy
   (d) streaks of chorioretinal atrophy in the peripheral fundus *curvi FAg*
     Rx. ?   Rx CNV — laser if leak away from curvi FAg

Congenital toxoplasmosis *esp 1st trimester*

Caused by infection of fetus with obligate intracellular protozoan parasite *Toxoplasma gondii*. Toxoplasmosis can also be acquired in adult life—an acute retinitis may occur.

1 General features:
   (a) prenatal death
   (b) CNS damage: *minority suffer from disseminated infection*
     (i) mentally handicapped
     (ii) convulsions
     (iii) hydrocephalus
     (iv) intracranial calcification
2 Ocular features: *Retina is only primary site of ocular infection with 2° affectn on nv, Choroid + ant seg*
   (a) anterior uveitis; may be granulomatous
   (b) vitritis
   (c) focal retinitis
   (d) juxtapapillary retinochoroiditis (Jensen's choroiditis)
   (e) optic neuritis
   (f) retinochoroidal scars

Toxocariasis

Caused by infection with *Toxocara canis* and *Toxocara catis*. Acquired by ingestion of ova. *in faces of dogs*

1 General features:
   (a) visceral larva migrans:
     (i) disseminated larvae
     (ii) fever
     (iii) lymphadenopathy
     (iv) hepatomegaly
     (v) pneumonitis
     (vi) eosinophilia
   (b) subclinical (most of the cases with ocular involvement have subclinical disease)
2 Ocular features: *in three forms*
   (a) peripheral retinal granuloma
   (b) localised posterior pole granuloma → *Choroid NV mem.*
   (c) chronic destructive endophthalmitis
   (d) virtually all cases unilateral

Onchocerciasis

As a result of infection with filarial nematode *Onchocerca volvulus*. An estimated 40 million people are affected (2 million blind). Transmitted by a black fly of genus *Simulium* which breeds in fast flowing rivers.

1 General features: skin nodules, lichenification, and depigmentation; large folds of skin ("hanging groins"); erysipelas-like or papular rash

2 Ocular features:
  (a) lids: skin nodules and depigmentation
  (b) cornea: sclerosing keratitis; microfilariae may occasionally be seen in the anterior chamber if patient has been in the dark
  (c) scleritis
  (d) chronic iridocyclitis
  (e) cataract and glaucoma
  (f) fundus: choroidoretinitis; optic atrophy (main cause of blindness)

SPECIFIC UVEITIS ENTITIES

Pars planitis
Usually affects young adults; both eyes involved in 80%; F > M.

1 Symptoms:
  (a) floaters
  (b) impaired vision

2 Signs:
  (a) light flare with a few keratic precipitates
  (b) anterior vitritis
  (c) white exudates near the ora serrata (snowballs); exudates may coalesce to form a snowbank
  (d) mild peripheral periphlebitis

3 Complications:
  (a) cataract
  (b) retrolenticular cyclitic membrane
  (c) neovascularisation and vitreous haemorrhage
  (d) tractional retinal detachment
  (e) macular oedema

4 Differential diagnosis:
  (a) sarcoidosis
  (b) toxoplasmosis
  (c) peripheral toxocariasis
  (d) syphilis
  (e) multiple sclerosis

Fuchs' heterochromic cyclitis

Affects one eye of young adults, but there may be bilaterality.

1 Symptoms: usually blurred vision from cataract or vitreous opacity

2 Signs:
  (a) small keratic precipitates diffusely spread throughout the endothelium
  (b) only a few cells and faint flare in the anterior chamber
  (c) no posterior synechiae
  (d) heterochromia
  (e) abnormal blood vessels in the anterior chamber angle which may bleed on gonioscopy and during surgery

    (f) secondary open angle glaucoma
    (g) posterior subcapsular cataract
3 Other causes of heterochromia:
    (a) idiopathic
    (b) inherited
    (c) trauma
    (d) inflammation
    (e) retained metallic intraocular foreign body
    (f) congenital Horner's syndrome
    (g) melanoma
    (h) Waardenberg's syndrome (heterochromia iridis, telecanthus, white forelock, and congenital deafness)
    (i) Parry–Romberg syndrome (heterochromia iridis, Horner's syndrome, oculomotor palsies, nystagmus, and facial hemiatrophy)
    (j) glaucomatocyclitic crisis

Vogt–Koyanagi–Harada syndrome *(autoimmune against melanocyte)*

Occurs between the ages of 30 and 50 years; rare, but occurs more commonly in Japanese, Middle Eastern and Asian patients.
1 Cutaneous features:
    (a) alopecia
    (b) vitiligo
    (c) whitening of eyelashes (poliosis) *prodromal stage - few days.*
2 CNS features:
    (a) meningeal irritation with headache and neck stiffness
    (b) encephalopathy with cranial nerve palsies and convulsions
    (c) vertigo, deafness, and tinnitus
3 Ocular features:
    (a) granulomatous anterior uveitis *Demicunati (similar to sym ophth.)*
    (b) multifocal choroiditis *acute uveitis stage*
    (c) bilateral exudative retinal detachments
    (d) vitritis *ocular [Chronic - depigment of Choroid + ciliary + hair + eyelash*
    (d) macular oedema
    (e) disc hyperaemia

Rx system steroid and/or cyclosporin

Sympathetic ophthalmia

Usually occurs in fellow eye following penetrating trauma; may also occur after cataract extraction and perforating corneal ulcers; occurs between 10 days and 50 years after injury.
1 Symptoms:
    (a) photophobia
    (b) red eye
    (c) blurring of vision *recurrent episodes are common.*
2 Signs:
    (a) ciliary flush
    (b) Koeppe's nodules on iris
    (c) posterior synechiae
    (d) large mutton fat keratic precipitates
    (e) subretinal oedema

Complication [Cataract, 2° glaucoma, optic atrophy, RD, iris neovas.

    (f) yellow–white subretinal spots (Dalen–Fuchs nodules) *RPE*
    (g) oedema optic disc
3 Histology:
    (a) panuveal cellular infiltration
    (b) pale islands of epithelioid macrophages and giant cells among hyperchromatic infiltrating lymphocytes
    (c) phagocytosed melanin in the cytoplasm of epithelioid and giant cells
    (d) Dalen–Fuchs nodules: nodules of ciliary epithelial cells and epithelioid macrophages beneath and between the pigmented and non-pigmented layers of the ciliary epithelium; these nodules are also found in ocular tuberculosis and Vogt–Koyanagi–Harada syndrome

Birdshot retinochoroidopathy

Present blurry of vision

Affects patients over the age of 40; increased incidence of HLA-A29; F > M.
1 Ocular features:

↓ night vis + Colon vis
ERG + EOG - abnormal

    (a) usually bilateral
    (b) mild anterior chamber activity
    (c) vitritis → *floaters*
    (d) chorioretinal lesions, depigmented spots at the level of the retinal pigment epithelium (RPE) *Creamy around ophthalmic disc → equator*
    (e) retinal vasculitis → *cmo*
    (f) subretinal neovascularisation
    (g) cystoid macular oedema
    (h) optic disc swelling → *atrophy*

Acute multifocal placoid pigment epitheliopathy (AMPPE)

Affects young adults; 'flu-like prodromal syndrome may occur.
1 Systemic features:
    (a) thyroiditis
    (b) erythema nodosum
    (c) cerebral vasculitis
    (d) regional enteritis
2 Ocular features:
    (a) usually affects both eyes
    (b) episcleritis
    (c) anterior uveitis
    (d) vitritis
    (e) cream coloured placoid areas which coalesce in the posterior pole of both eyes
    (f) vascular sheathing and disc oedema may occur

Serpiginous choroidopathy

Affects patients between 40 and 60 years of age.
Ocular features:
    (a) usually bilateral but asymmetrical

   (b) mild anterior uveitis
   (c) vitritis
   (d) cream coloured chorioretinal lesions (at RPE level) with hazy borders starting around the optic disc; recurrent attacks with spread of the lesions peripherally in all directions
   (e) subretinal neovascularisation may occur

Acute retinal necrosis (ARN) *most Commonly Caused by HS, H2*

Usually affects young patients; bilateral in 30–50% of cases.
1 Ocular features:
   (a) present with acute visual loss (*ophi neuritis*)
   (b) mild anterior uveitis
   (c) vitritis; may lead to tractional retinal detachment (much less common than rhegmatogenous detachment)
   (d) full thickness necrosis of the retina beginning at the periphery and spreading centrally
   (e) retinal holes (70%); may lead to retinal detachment

HLA associations in uveitis

1 Ankylosing spondylitis—HLA-B27
2 Reiter's syndrome—HLA-B27
3 Behçet's syndrome—HLA-B5 (Japanese)
4 Vogt–Koyanagi–Harada syndrome—HLA-B22, HLA-BW54, HLA-DR4MT3
5 Sympathetic ophthalmia—HLA-A11
6 Birdshot retinochoroidopathy—HLA-A29
7 Presumed ocular histoplasmosis—HLA-B7

*See page 239. Syphium HLA**

Management of uveitis

Exact management will depend on type of uveitis.
1 Exclude and treat any underlying cause, e.g. syphilitic uveitis
2 Exclude and treat complications, e.g. glaucoma
3 Steroids: route:
   (a) topical
   (b) subconjunctival
   (c) periocular
   (d) systemic
4 Mydriatics:
   (a) route:
      (i) topical
      (ii) subconjunctival
   (b) indication:
      (i) prevent synechiae
      (ii) reduce ciliary spasm
      (iii) (reduce vascular permeability, particularly atropine)
5 Immunosuppressants, e.g. azathioprine, cyclosporin

ENDOPHTHALMITIS

Inflammation of one or more coats of the eye and adjacent intraocular spaces. Clinically used to describe potentially destructive inflammation in the retina, choroid, and adjacent intraocular spaces.

Types

1 Infectious:
  (a) exogenous, e.g. secondary to intraocular surgery
  (b) endogenous, e.g. secondary to bacterial carditis
2 Non-infectious:
  (a) lens induced
  (b) foreign bodies, e.g. copper and ophthalmia nodosa from caterpillar hairs

Symptoms

1 Pain
2 Decreased visual acuity
3 Ocular discharge
4 Headache
5 Red eye
6 Photophobia

Signs

1 Eyelid swelling
2 Red eye
3 Conjunctival oedema (chemosis)
4 White cells in anterior chamber settling as a hypopyon
5 Fibrin in anterior chamber
6 Vitreous activity and decreased red reflex "puff-balls" in the vitreous cavity
7 Retinal haemorrhages
8 White plaque in capsule suggests *Propionibacterium acnes* post cataract endophthalmitis

Causes of endophthalmitis after intraocular surgery

1 Gram positive bacteria (90%):
  (a) *Staphylococcus epidermidis* (20–50%) ⎫
  (b) *Staphylococcus aureus* ⎪
  (c) *Streptococcus pneumoniae* ⎪
  (d) *Streptococcus viridans* ⎬ Aerobic
  (e) *Streptococcus pyogenes* ⎪
  (f) *Corynebacterium* spp. ⎭
  (g) *Peptostreptococcus* spp. ⎫
  (h) *Propionibacterium acnes* ⎬ Anaerobic
  (i) *Clostridium* spp. ⎭
2 Gram negative bacteria (7%):
  (a) *Pseudomonas aeruginosa*
  (b) *Proteus* spp.
  (c) *Haemophilus influenzae*

91

   (d) *Klebsiella pneumoniae*
   (e) *Escherichia coli*
   (f) *Enterobacter aerogenes*
3 Fungi (3%): present later (one or more weeks):
   (a) *Aspergillus* spp.
   (b) *Candida* spp.
   (c) *Cephalosporium* spp.
   (d) *Paecilomyces* spp.
   (e) *Penicillium* spp.

Most common infecting organisms after glaucoma filtering surgery

1 Streptococci (57%)
2 *Haemophilus influenzae* (23%)
3 *Staphylococcus aureus*

Causes of endogenous endophthalmitis

1 Fungal:
   (a) *Candida albicans* (75–80% of all endogenous endophthalmitis)
   (b) *Aspergillus* spp.
2 Bacterial:
   (a) *Neisseria meningitidis*
   (b) *Streptococcus* spp.
   (c) *Staphylococcus aureus*
   (d) *Bacillus cereus*
   (e) *Nocardia asteroides*

Management of endophthalmitis

Exact details depend on type and circumstances of endophthalmitis.
1 Diagnosis:
   (a) clinical features
   (b) anterior chamber and vitreous tap:
      (i) Gram and Giemsa stains
      (ii) centrifuge vitreous to concentrate organisms or filter
      (iii) blood agar
      (iv) chocolate agar
      (v) cooked meat broth   } media
      (vi) Sabouraud's
      (vii) liaise with microbiologist
   (c) blood culture in endogenous cases
2 Treatment:
   (a) antibiotics:
      (i) topical (intensive and high concentration)
      (ii) subconjunctival
      (iii) intraocular—low volume, exact dose, no preservatives
      (iv) systemic
   (b) vitrectomy
   (c) steroids:
      (i) topical
      (ii) systemic

7
THE GLAUCOMAS

Definition: a group of conditions with a characteristic optic neuropathy in which the intraocular pressure is sufficiently raised to impair normal function of the optic nerve.

THE CILIARY BODY

1 Anatomy:
   (a) triangular in cross section, extending from ora serrata to scleral spur 6 mm in width
   (b) anterior surface: shortest; uveal portion of the trabecular meshwork
   (c) outer surface: lies against sclera; lines potential suprachoroidal space
   (d) inner surface: posterior $\frac{2}{3}$ is the pars plana; anterior $\frac{1}{3}$ is the pars plicata; pars plicata has 70 ciliary processes 0·8 mm high, 1 mm wide
2 Histology:
   (a) uveal portion:
      (i) ciliary muscle (unstriated); three components: longitudinal bundle, radial bundle, and circular bundle
      (ii) layer of vessels from major circle of iris (ciliary loops)
      (iii) basal lamina continuous with Bruch's membrane
   (b) epithelial:
      (i) inner, non-pigmented epithelium portion equivalent to sensory retina; basal lamina continuous with internal limiting membrane of retina
      (ii) outer pigmented epithelium equivalent to retinal pigment epithelium; zonula occludens present; basal lamina continuous with cuticular layer of Bruch's membrane
3 Blood supply: major circle of iris from 2 long ciliary arteries, 7 anterior ciliary arteries
4 Nerve supply:
   (a) ciliary muscle: postganglionic parasympathetic fibres from oculomotor nerve via short ciliary nerves
   (b) blood vessels: sympathetic fibres also via short ciliary nerves
5 Functions:
   (a) aqueous humour formation:

      (i) ultrafiltration
      (ii) active secretion
  (b) accommodation
  (c) control of aqueous outflow
  (d) secretion of hyaluronic acid into the vitreous
  (e) blood–aqueous barrier
6 Embryology:
  (a) formed by fusion of optic cup (neuroectoderm) and surrounding mesoderm
  (b) ciliary processes formed from epithelium of developing retina
  (c) ciliary muscle formed from mesoderm; longitudinal fibres formed by 4 months; circular fibres formed by 6 months
  (d) aqueous circulation starts at 6–7 months

TRABECULAR MESHWORK

Encircles the circumference of the anterior chamber.
1 Uveal meshwork: cord shaped collagenous core surrounded by endothelial cells; openings up to 70 μm in diameter; linked to ciliary muscle
2 Corneoscleral meshwork: sheet like beams insert into scleral spur; openings up to 30 μm in diameter
3 Juxtacanalicular tissue: links corneoscleral trabeculae with canal of Schlemm endothelium; trabecular organisation absent; openings 4–7 μm in width

CANAL OF SCHLEMM

1 Oval channel encircling circumference of the anterior chamber
2 Inner surface is in contact with juxtacanalicular tissue
3 Outer surface buried in corneoscleral stroma
4 Lined with single layer of endothelial cells
5 Passage of aqueous from trabecular meshwork to canal is controversial; possibilities:
  (a) leaky endothelial cell junctions
  (b) transcellular channels
  (c) giant vacuoles (pinocytosis)
6 Canal connects with the venous system by 25–35 collector channels

AQUEOUS DRAINAGE

1 Conventional route: intraocular pressure dependent; drains to canal of Schlemm, then deep scleral plexus into anterior ciliary and episcleral veins or into conjunctival aqueous veins
2 Uveoscleral route: intraocular pressure independent; drains via anterior ciliary body face to suprachoroidal space, then to uveal or vortex veins or trans-sclerally to orbital veins

FEATURES OF THE ANTERIOR CHAMBER ANGLE (ON GONIOSCOPY)

1 Schwalbe's line: seen anteriorly; peripheral termination of Descemet's membrane; prominent and anterior in 15% of normal eyes (posterior embryotoxon)
2 Trabecular meshwork: from Schwalbe's line to scleral spur; more pigmented posteriorly
3 Schlemm's canal: sometimes seen in posterior trabeculum, especially if filled with blood
4 Scleral spur: most anterior part of sclera; site of attachment of longitudinal bundle of ciliary muscle
5 Ciliary body: brown band just behind scleral spur
6 Peripheral iris
7 Iris processes: insert from iris to scleral spur; more prominent in childhood
8 Iris blood vessels: circular are most common; radial are rarer

Angle width grading (Scheie)

1 Grade 4: widest angle opening (35–45°):
   (a) ciliary body easily seen
   (b) seen in high myopia and aphakia
   (c) closure impossible
2 Grade 3: scleral spur visible:
   (a) closure impossible
3 Grade 2: trabecular meshwork seen:
   (a) angle closure possible but unlikely
4 Grade 1: Schwalbe's line and top of trabecular meshwork seen:
   (a) high angle closure risk
5 Grade 0: iridocorneal contact:
   (a) complete closed angle

Abnormal gonioscopic findings

1 Blood in canal of Schlemm:
   (a) secondary to gonioscopy
   (b) carotid–cavernous fistula
   (c) superior vena cava obstruction
   (d) Sturge–Weber syndrome
   (e) ocular hypotony
2 Abnormal angle blood vessels:
   (a) neovascular glaucoma
   (b) anterior uveitis
   (c) Fuchs' heterochromic cyclitis
3 Hyperpigmented angle:
   (a) pigment dispersion syndrome
   (b) pseudoexfoliation syndrome
   (c) laser iridotomy
   (d) anterior segment surgery
   (e) longstanding iritis

   (f) trauma
   (g) melanoma
   (h) increasing age
4 Peripheral anterior synechiae:
   (a) angle closure
   (b) uveitis
   (c) neovascularisation
   (d) loss of anterior chamber
   (e) iris bombé
   (f) essential iris atrophy
   (g) tumour of ciliary body
   (h) cleavage syndromes

AQUEOUS HUMOUR

1 Fills anterior and posterior chamber
2 Volume of anterior chamber aqueous: 0·25 ml
3 Volume of posterior chamber aqueous: 0·06 ml
4 Refractive index: 1·336
5 Production rate: 2–3 μl/min
6 Drainage rate:
   (a) 2 μl/min, conventional route
   (b) 0·2 μl/min, uveoscleral route
7 Composition varies between posterior and anterior chambers
   (a) $[Na^+]$ $\left.\right\}$ lower in posterior chamber
   (b) $[Cl^-]$
   (c) $[PO_4^{3-}]$ $\left.\right\}$ higher in posterior chamber
   (d) $[HCO_3^-]$

INTRAOCULAR PRESSURE

1 Dependent on balance between inflow and outflow of aqueous humour
2 Intraocular pressure in UK: average 16·5 mm Hg; standard deviation 2·5 mm Hg; distribution skewed slightly towards higher pressures
3 Variation of 1-2 mm Hg with heartbeat and respiration
4 Diurnal variation of 2–3 mm Hg; highest on awakening, lowest during evening
5 Increases transiently on lying down and the Valsalva manoeuvre

Measurement of intraocular pressure

1 Indentation tonometry: plunger indents a soft eye more than a hard eye:
   (a) Schiötz tonometer: scleral rigidity affects accuracy of measurement; underestimation if rigidity low, e.g. myopia, dysthyroid disease, miotic treatment
   (b) pneumotonometer: detects change of gas flow through a flexible diaphragm

2 Applanation: relies on application of Imbert–Fick principle (the tonometry force required to flatten an area of a sphere is proportional to the pressure within the sphere):
   (a) Goldmann tonometer: when the flattened area is 3·06 mm the surface tension of tears balances the elastic force of the cornea; gram force $\times$ 10 is directly convertible into mm Hg
   (b) Mackay–Marg: partly applanation, partly indentation tonometer; 1·5 mm plunger protruding 5 µm beyond surface footplate; can be used on scarred, irregular corneas; Tonopen uses same principle
   (c) non-contact: uses an air puff to flatten cornea; light tonometer reflected from flattened corneal surface to photoreceptor; tends to overestimate intraocular pressure, especially in higher ranges

PRIMARY OPEN ANGLE GLAUCOMA

Affects 1 in 200 of population over 40 years of age; responsible for around 15% of blind registrations in the UK.
1 Pathogenesis: histological features include:
   (a) trabecular:
      (i) endothelial cell loss meshwork
      (ii) alterations to extracellular matrix
      (iii) loss of giant vacuoles from canal of Schlemm
      (iv) increase in trabecular thickness
      (v) excessive fusion of trabeculae
      (vi) hyperpigmentation of meshwork cells
   (b) optic disc:
      (i) compression and collapse of lamina cribrosa collagen bundles
      (ii) swollen axons at optic nerve head with hold up of axoplasmic transport
      (iii) eventual selective axonal destruction in "hour glass" pattern at optic disc
         (changes in the trabecular meshwork may impede aqueous outflow, and thus increase intraocular pressure)
   (c) visual loss may occur by:
      (i) direct mechanical effects on nerve fibres
      (ii) vascular insufficiency to optic nerve head
         (characteristic pattern of nerve loss may relate to regional differences in axonal support, lamina cribrosa, or vascular supply to optic nerve head)
      (iii) ganglion cell death. May be a component of apoptosis (programmed cell death)
2 Criteria for diagnosis:
   (a) glaucomatous cupping of the optic disc
   (b) glaucomatous visual field defect
   (c) open angle on gonioscopy
   (d) (intraocular pressure >21 mm Hg) (note that concepts are changing; there is no absolute pressure definition)
3 Optic disc changes:
   (a) cup/disc (C/D) ratio:

       (i) normal <0·3 but increases with age, varies, dependent on the area of the scleral canal. Afro-Caribbeans have larger C/D ratios

       (ii) asymmetry of >0·2 is suspicious

       (iii) notching of rim is suspicious

   (b) pallor: area of disc lacking small vessels; no increase with age

   (c) nasal shift of blood vessels at the disc and "undermining" of vessels

   (d) haemorrhages on the disc or disc margin

   (e) retinal nerve fibre layer atrophy: visible in red free light

   (f) difficulties arise in:

       (i) high myopia

       (ii) congenital disc anomalies

       (iii) media opacities

       (iv) small pupils

4 Visual field:

   (a) paracentral scotoma 10–20° from the blind spot

   (b) arcuate scotoma (Seidel's scotoma)

   (c) arcuate scotoma with breakthrough to the periphery

   (d) nasal step (Roenne's scotoma)

   (e) temporal wedge

   (f) generalised constriction often with residual island

   (g) kinetic:

       (i) Bjerrum screen—central 30° only testing

       (ii) Lister perimeter—peripheral fields only

       (iii) Goldmann perimeter—evaluates whole field

   (h) static:

       (i) adapted Goldmann perimeter

       (ii) Friedmann perimeter

       (iii) computer assisted—automatically test suprathreshold and threshold stimuli, and quantify depth of field defect

5 Associations:

   (a) ocular:

       (i) high myopia

       (ii) retinal vein occlusion

       (iii) retinal detachment

       (iv) Fuchs' endothelial dystrophy

       (v) retinitis pigmentosa

   (b) systemic: diabetes mellitus

   (c) (after 40) family history: direct relatives of sufferers have about an 8% chance (1 in 12) of developing disease; annual screening by optometrist recommended

   (d) increasing age

Methods of assessing ocular blood flow

1 Fluorescein angiography
2 Indocynanine green angiography (better for choroid)
3 Pulsatile ocular blood flow
4 Laser Doppler velocimeter (surface disc flow)
5 Heidelberg retinal flowmeter

Treatment of primary open angle glaucoma

1 Medical:
   (a) topical:
      (i) β-blockers
      (ii) miotics
      (iii) sympathomimetics
      (iv) carbonic anhydrase inhibitors
      (v) α-antagonists
      (vi) prostaglandin analogues
   (b) systemic: carbonic anhydrase inhibitors
2 Surgical:
   (a) argon laser trabeculoplasty
   (b) drainage surgery
   (c) cyclodestructive procedure

Laser trabeculoplasty

1 Indications:
   (a) elderly patients: poorly controlled and unable to tolerate surgery; previously:
      (i) visual field loss continuing on maximum tolerated medical therapy
      (ii) high intraocular pressure uncontrolled by drugs
      (iii) poor compliance with medical therapy
      (iv) replacement of poorly tolerated medication
      (v) medically unfit for glaucoma surgery
2 Mechanism:
   (a) uncertain
   (b) cellular: regeneration of trabecular meshwork cells
   (c) biochemical: new type of extracellular matrix
   (d) mechanical: collagen shrinkage
3 Good response:
   (a) primary open angle glaucoma
   (b) pseudoexfoliative glaucoma
   (c) pigmentary glaucoma
4 Poor response:
   (a) steroid induced glaucoma
   (b) ghost cell glaucoma
   (c) uveitic glaucoma
   (d) juvenile open angle glaucoma
   (e) iridocorneal endothelial syndrome
   (f) iridocorneal mesodermal dysgenesis
   (g) glaucoma caused by elevated episcleral venous pressure
   (h) aphakic glaucoma
   (i) angle recession glaucoma
5 Technique:
   (a) power: 700–1500 mW
   (b) 50 μm spot size
   (c) 0·1 second, 50 burns; 180° less complications than 360°
   (d) depigmentation spot

   (e) variety of lasers can be used, most commonly argon, but diode, krypton, and neodymium:yttrium–aluminium–garnet (Nd:YAG; free running) also used; diode may cause less inflammation
6 Complications:
   (a) transient rise of intraocular pressure
   (b) persistent rise of intraocular pressure
   (c) transient blurring of vision
   (d) worsening of visual field defects
   (e) anterior uveitis
   (f) peripheral anterior synechiae
   (g) ?long term effects on meshwork and subsequent surgery
7 Results:
   (a) reduction of intraocular pressure (IOP) by 6-9 mm Hg
   (b) loss of IOP control in 10% of patients per year

Glaucoma filtering surgery

1 Indications:
   (a) as a primary treatment
   (b) if no response to minimal medical therapy; previously:
       (i) continuing visual field loss on maximum tolerated medical therapy
       (ii) high intraocular pressure uncontrolled by drugs
       (iii) poor compliance of medical therapy
       (iv) poor response after argon laser trabeculoplasty
2 High risk failure:
   (a) previous failed trabeculectomy
   (b) previous conjunctival surgery/incision, including cataract surgery
   (c) children
   (d) Afro-Caribbean patients
   (e) aphakic individuals
   (f) neovascular glaucoma
   (g) previous medical therapy (especially adrenaline)
   (h) inflammation (uveitis)
   (i) multiple previous episodes of intraocular surgery
3 Healing response:
   (a) incision
   (b) blood release including growth factors
   (c) clotting with fibrin/fibronectin matrix
   (d) inflammatory cell response
   (e) fibroblast proliferation/synthesis remodelling of matrix
   (f) final scar
4 Modulation of healing response:
   (a) surgical technique
   (b) fibrinolytics, e.g. tissue plasminogen activator
   (c) steroids
   (d) anti-proliferative agents, e.g. 5-fluorouracil (5-FU), mitomycin C (MMC), β-radiation
       (i) injections or single dose regimens based on laboratory studies, e.g. Moorfields/Florida titratable regimen

    (ii) low risk—nothing or 5-FU 25 mg/ml for 5 min
   (iii) medium risk—5-FU 25 mg/ml or MMC 0·2 mg/ml for 5 min
   (iv) high risk—MMC 0·4 mg/ml (thick tissues) for 5 min
    (v) note the full cytotoxic handling precautions—must be washed out before eye is entered
   (vi) potential risks: tissue damage including endothelium/bleb leaks/hypotony, and effusions and maculopathy/scleromalacia/ ?endophthalmitis risk
  (e) anti-collagen cross linking agents, e.g. β-aminopropionitrile
5 Possible mechanisms of pressure lowering:
  (a) outflow via blood vessels (old and newly formed)
  (b) outflow via lymphatics
  (c) transconjunctival outflow (especially thin blebs)
  (d) (via open Schlemm's canal)
  (e) inadvertent cyclodialysis
6 Complications:
  (a) flat anterior chamber
  (b) hypotony
  (c) choroidal detachments and folds
  (d) hyphaema
  (e) malignant (ciliary block) glaucoma
  (f) cataract formation (10%)
  (g) visual field deterioration
  (h) endophthalmitis (early or late)
  (i) bleb failure
  (j) maculopathy (particularly myopic individuals)

Other procedures

Implant (Seton/tube)
1 Principle: tube to maintain flow path and plate of variable area providing an aqueous reservoir, e.g. Molteno, Schocket, Joseph, with or without a valve or flow restricting device

Cyclodestructive procedure
1 Principle: destruction of ciliary processes and aqueous production
2 Methods: cryotherapy (quick freeze–slow thaw), Nd–YAG (free running mode), or diode laser both delivered on slitlamp or via trans-scleral contact probe; in theory contact Nd–YAG and diode laser superior as minimal damage to conjunctiva and sclera

ACUTE ANGLE CLOSURE GLAUCOMA

1 Incidence:
  (a) 1 in 1000 people over 40 years
  (b) M:F = 1:4
2 Symptoms:
  (a) pain
  (b) coloured haloes
  (c) headache
  (d) nausea, vomiting

    (e) previous history of subacute attacks
3 Signs:
    (a) reduced vision
    (b) ciliary injection
    (c) corneal oedema
    (d) mid-dilated vertically oval pupil
    (e) shallow anterior chamber
    (f) flare and cells in anterior chamber
    (g) congested iris vessels
    (h) iris stromal oedema
    (i) central retinal artery pulsation
4 Predisposing factors:
    (a) hypermetropia
    (b) small corneal diameter
    (c) short axial length of globe
    (d) large crystalline lens
    (e) shallow anterior chamber (<2·5 mm)
5 Provocative tests: used in latent or subacute cases; positive result if 8 mm Hg pressure rise occurs in 1 hour; types:
    (a) physiological:
        (i) dark room test
        (ii) prone test
        (iii) prone dark room test (patient must remain awake)
    (b) pharmacological:
        (i) 10% phenylephrine (reversible with thymoxamine)
        (ii) 10% phenylephrine and 2% pilocarpine
6 Sequelae:
    (a) poor vision
    (b) sectorial iris atrophy
    (c) spiralling of iris fibres
    (d) iris hole (pseudopolycoria)
    (e) large irregular pupil
    (f) *glaukomflecken*
    (g) peripheral anterior synechiae
    (h) chronic corneal oedema
7 Treatment:
    (a) initial:
        (i) acetazolamide 500 mg i.v., then 250 mg p.o. 4 times a day
        (ii) pilocarpine 4% every 15 minutes for 1 hour, then 4 times a day; note the poor penetration when IOP is raised, and the potential systemic toxicity
        (iii) topical steroids
        (iv) β blockers
        (v) if no response osmotic agents, e.g. glycerol 1–2 g/kg body weight p.o. in lemon juice and/or mannitol 1–2 g/kg body weight (20% solution) given i.v. over 30 min
        (vi) occasional corneal indentation
        (vii) treat pain and nausea
    (b) late:
        (i) medical therapy if infirm

    (ii) surgery—peripheral iridectomy; laser iridotomy; filtration surgery; iridectomy/iridotomy on fellow eye

CHRONIC CLOSED ANGLE GLAUCOMA

1 Clinical features:
    (a) painless
    (b) angle partially closed
    (c) peripheral anterior synechiae
    (d) intraocular pressure mildly elevated
    (e) visual field defects
2 Treatment: depends on degree of peripheral anterior synechiae:
    (a) medical
    (b) surgical: peripheral iridectomy; laser iridotomy; filtration surgery

SECONDARY OPEN ANGLE GLAUCOMA

1 Pre-trabecular: membrane preventing access to angle:
    (a) fibrovascular membrane (neovascularisation)
    (b) endothelial membrane (iridocorneal endothelial syndrome):
        (i) Cogan–Reese syndrome (iris naevus)
        (ii) Chandler's syndrome
        (iii) essential iris atrophy
    (c) epithelial downgrowth
    (d) fibrous ingrowth
2 Trabecular:
    (a) clogging of meshwork:
        (i) red blood cells—hyphaema; ghost cell glaucoma
        (ii) macrophages—haemolytic; phakoanaphylactic; melanomyelocytic
        (iii) neoplastic cells—malignant tumours; neurofibromatosis; juvenile xanthogranuloma
        (iv) pigment—pigmentary glaucoma; pseudoexfoliation; long-standing uveitis; malignant melanoma
        (v) protein—uveitis; lens induced
        (vi) α-chymotrypsin induced
        (vii) vitreous disruption
        (viii) pseudoexfoliative material
    (b) alteration of meshwork:
        (i) oedema—uveitis; scleritis; alkali burns
        (ii) trauma—angle recession
        (iii) intraocular foreign body—haemosiderosis and chalcosis
        (iv) steroid induced
3 Post-trabecular: high episcleral venous pressure preventing outflow:
    (a) carotid–cavernous fistula
    (b) cavernous sinus thrombosis
    (c) orbital tumours
    (d) dysthyroid eye disease
    (e) superior vena cava obstruction

(f) mediastinal tumours
(g) Sturge–Weber syndrome
(h) idiopathic

SECONDARY CLOSED ANGLE GLAUCOMA

1 With pupil block:
  (a) intumescent lens
  (b) subluxation of lens
  (c) following lens extraction
  (d) pseudophakia, especially intracapsular lens extraction and anterior chamber implant
  (e) iris bombé caused by ring synechiae
2 Without pupil block:
  (a) malignant (ciliary block) glaucoma
  (b) following scleral buckling
  (c) following panretinal photocoagulation
  (d) intraocular tumours
  (e) cysts of iris and ciliary body
  (f) retrolental tissue contraction:
      (i) retinopathy of prematurity
      (ii) persistent hyperplastic primary vitreous

LENS INDUCED GLAUCOMAS

1 Phakomorphic: causes pupil block and secondary angle closure by:
  (a) lens intumescence
  (b) lens dislocation (anteriorly and posteriorly)
2 Phakolytic: leak of lens proteins; clogs trabecular meshwork
3 Phakoanaphylactic: sensitisation of eye or its fellow to lens protein; inflammatory material clogs trabecular meshwork

PSEUDOEXFOLIATION SYNDROME

Presence of widely dispersed abnormal amyloid like deposits; more common in Scandinavians. Bilateral asymmetrical condition, often more advanced in one eye; 70% associated with raised intraocular pressure.
1 Features:
  (a) flakes of material seen on:
      (i) anterior lens capsule
      (ii) pupil margin
      (iii) ciliary processes
      (iv) zonule
      (v) anterior hyaloid face
  (b) pigmented trabecular meshwork
  (c) pigment on Schwalbe's line (Sampaolesi's line); treatment of glaucoma is difficult

PIGMENT DISPERSION SYNDROME

Bilateral disorder; uncommon in Afro-Caribbeans; often affects myopic young men; IOP may rise after exercise.
1 Features:
    (a) radial iris transillumination in midperiphery
    (b) pigment loss from posterior iris pigment epithelium
    (c) pigment deposited on:
        (i) corneal endothelium (Krukenberg's spindle)
        (ii) trabecular meshwork
        (iii) Schwalbe's line (Sampaolesi's line)
        (iv) lens
        (v) zonule
        (vi) iris
    (d) deep anterior chamber (possibly resulting from "reverse" pupil block); peripheral iridectomy may alter iris profile and stop iris chafing

CAUSES OF INCREASED IOP IN UVEITIS

1 Mechanical blockage of molecular meshwork by serum components as a result of blood–aqueous barrier breakdown
2 Hypertension associated with prostaglandin mediated vascular hyperpermeability
3 Over taxing of outflow mechanisms by protein that interferes with active transport
4 Inflammation of the trabecular meshwork itself with swelling that causes outflow
5 Damage to trabecular endothelial cells by the inflammatory process
6 Mechanical obstruction of outflow by precipitates on the meshwork
7 Sclerosis of trabecular meshwork as a result of chronic inflammation
8 Obstruction of the trabecular hyaline membrane
9 Secondary to steroid treatment

NEOVASCULAR GLAUCOMA

Presence of glaucoma with a fibrovascular membrane occluding the drainage angle. First described by Coats in 1906.
1 Pathogenesis:
    (a) stimulus to new vessel formation usually related to posterior segment ischaemia
    (b) release of peptide growth factors that diffuse to the front of the eye and stimulate new vessel formation; inhibitors of neovascularisation may be secreted by cells in the normal eye; e.g. retinal pigment epithelium; these inhibitors may be reduced in neovascular glaucoma
    (c) proliferation begins at pupil margin and spreads centrifugally
    (d) progressive peripheral anterior synechiae result in angle closure
2 Causes:
    (a) vascular:

(i) retinal vein occlusion: 30 + % of cases; up to 20% of patients with CRVO develop rubeosis; correlated with retinal non-perfusion; incidence 60% when ischaemia present on fluorescein, 1% of eyes with good capillary perfusion; predictive tests include relative afferent pupillary defect, ERG Cb wag delay and reduced b wave/a wave ratio
(ii) diabetic retinopathy: 30 + % of cases
(iii) retinal artery occlusion
(iv) carotid artery occlusive disease
(v) retinopathy
(b) inflammatory:
    (i) chronic uveitis
    (ii) endophthalmitis
    (iii) sympathetic ophthalmia
    (iv) longstanding retinal detachment
(c) neoplastic:
    (i) retinoblastoma
    (ii) choroidal malignant melanoma
    (iii) choroidal metastases
(d) surgical:
    (i) cataract extraction (especially if capsule removed)
    (ii) vitrectomy—20–40% incidence after pars plana vitrectomy in diabetic patients; highest incidence within 6 months of vitrectomy; reduced with silicone oil; ?barrier function
    (iii) retinal detachment surgery—successful surgery may lead to regression of neovascularisation
3 Treatment:
(a) removal of stimulus, e.g. retinal panphotocoagulation (pupillary, trans-scleral, or endophotocoagulation); urgent or rubeotic angle changes may be irreversible
(b) medical management: avoid miotics e.g. pilocarpine
(c) cyclodestructive procedures
(d) glaucoma implants, e.g. Molteno tube
(e) filtration surgery: unassisted surgery doomed to failure; combine with anti-proliferative agent
(f) palliation:
    (i) topical atropine and steroids
    (ii) retrobulbar alcohol
    (iii) enucleation

PRIMARY CONGENITAL GLAUCOMA

Sporadic/autosomal recessive; affects 1 in 10 000 live births; M:F = 3:1; may be manifest at birth or develop later.
1 Features:
(a) lacrimation
(b) photophobia
(c) eye rubbing
(d) buphthalmos (with early onset):
    (i) corneal diameter >13 mm

    (ii) corneal oedema
    (iii) "healed" splits in Descemet's membrane—Haab's striae; virtually diagnostic but not always present
  (e) myopia (particularly if rapidly progressive)
  (f) variable optic disc cupping; most Caucasian children have C/D ratios <0·3
2 Gonioscopic findings:
  (a) Barkan's membrane (controversial)
  (b) thickening of trabecular sheets
  (c) insertion of iris above scleral spur
  (d) peripheral iris stroma hypoplasia

Differential diagnosis of cloudy cornea at birth

1 Glaucoma, primary or secondary
2 Trauma
3 Rubella and other intrauterine infections
4 Mucopolysaccharidoses
5 Mucolipidoses
6 Peters' anomaly
7 Corneal dystrophy

CAUSES OF SECONDARY CONGENITAL GLAUCOMA (AND PERCENTAGE WITH GLAUCOMA)

1 Rubella (10%)
2 Aniridia (50%)
3 Microcornea (60% closed angle)
4 Neurofibromatosis (25%)
5 Sturge–Weber syndrome (50%)
6 "Dysgenesis" syndromes (50%)
7 Lowe's syndrome (50%)

Aniridia (sporadic or autosomal dominant)

1 Features:
  (a) poor vision
  (b) nystagmus
  (c) photophobia
  (d) complete or partial absence of iris
  (e) angle anomalies
  (f) glaucoma—50%
  (g) corneal pannus
  (h) epibulbar dermoids
  (i) cataract
  (j) lens subluxation
  (k) hypoplastic macula

    (l) hypoplastic optic disc
  (m) Wilms' tumour in 20% of sporadic cases

Anterior segment dysgenesis

These are all probably a spectrum of diseases thought to be possibly associated with abnormalities of neural crest development. Primary congenital glaucoma may be part of this spectrum.

1 Axenfeld/Riegers (autosomal dominant) (iridiotrabeculodysgenesis):
  (a) only features:
       (i)   posterior embryotoxon
      (ii) iris strands to Schwalbe's line
     (iii) peripheral anterior synechial
     (iv) pupillary distortion   ⎫
      (v) peripheral corneal opacification ⎬ features described
     (vi) ectropion uveae   ⎭ by Rieger
    (vii) glaucoma in about 50% of cases
  (b) systemic features:
       (i)   abnormal dentition—reduced crown size (microdontia), reduced number of teeth (hypodontia), absence of teeth (anodontia)
      (ii) maxillary hypoplasia
     (iii) hypertelorism, telecanthus, micrognathia
     (iv) rare—empty sellar syndrome/growth hormone deficiency/heart defects; mental handicap; redundant periumbilical skin

2 Peters' anomaly:
  (a) 80% bilateral
  (b) associated with central defect of Descemet's membrane
  (c) types:
       (i)   central posterior corneal stromal opacity
      (ii) posterior stromal opacity with iris adhesions
     (iii) posterior corneal defect with lens adhesions
  (d) glaucoma in 50% of cases
  (e) corneal opacity may clear with pressure reduction
  (f) optical iridectomy may be indicated

Management of the developmental glaucomas

1 Intraocular pressure:
  (a) goniotomy for primary congenital glaucoma (clear cornea with alcohol)
  (b) trabeculotomy (if a/c not visible or Axenfeld/Riegers and Peters' group)
  (c) filtration surgery
      (with antifibrosis treatment, β radiation "rice regimen" at Moorfields)
  (d) cyclodestruction (cryotherapy now superseded by diode laser, but effects relatively temporary)
  (e) tube surgery

Need regular follow up for life (recurrence rate of about 2% per year even after successful treatment)

2 Treatment of associated ocular abnormalities; poor prognosis for corneal grafting
3 Management of whole family/future education, etc
4 Correction of refractive errors
5 Treatment of amblyopia

8
LENS

MACROSCOPIC ANATOMY

1 Biconvex, transparent
2 Diameter 10 mm
3 Thickness 4 mm
4 Anterior face radius 10 mm
5 Posterior face radius 6 mm

RELATIONS OF THE LENS

1 Anteriorly: iris and pupil
2 Posteriorly: patella fossa of anterior vitreous face
3 Surround: lens equator 0·5 mm from ciliary body

MICROSCOPIC ANATOMY

1 Lens capsule:
  (a) basement membrane of lens epithelium
  (b) smooth, acellular, elastic
  (c) composed of collagen and acid mucopolysaccharides
  (d) thickest distal to zonule insertion in midperiphery
2 Lens zonule (of Zinn):
  (a) suspensory ligament of lens
  (b) composed of fibrillin proteins
  (c) origin: from pigmented layer of ciliary body epithelium, from sides of processes and valleys; extending to pars plana
  (d) insertion: posterior fibres insert anteriorly 1 mm below equator; anterior fibres insert posteriorly 0·5 mm below equator; these two groups are separated by Petit's canal; form fine indentations in lens surface
3 Anterior lens epithelium: single cuboidal layer under anterior lens capsule

4 Lens fibres:
  (a) roughly hexagonal in cross section
  (b) 2100–2300 fibres; each fibre is a single cell
  (c) dimensions:
      (i) 7–10 μm long
      (ii) 7 μm wide in cortical zone, 5 μm in nuclear zone, and 2 μm near sutures
  (d) produced throughout life
  (e) cell division at lens equator
  (f) fibres elongate but initially have contact with epithelium and lens capsule
  (g) nuclei predominantly in equatorial zone
  (h) fibres shed towards lens centre
  (i) parallel to curved lens surface
  (j) radially placed
  (k) relatively few organelles, small nuclei
  (l) intracellular substance joining cells at sutures
  (m) fetal suture:
      (i) anteriorly Y shaped
      (ii) posteriorly Λ shaped
  (n) postfetal sutures increasingly complex
  (o) old fibres:
      (i) compressed centrally and lose nuclei
      (ii) form lens nucleus
5 Lens zone: concentric areas of differing refractive index:
  (a) subcapsular zone: clear
  (b) cortical zone: newly formed fibres
  (c) nuclear zone: old dense central fibres:
      (i) embryonic
      (ii) fetal
      (iii) infantile
      (iv) adult

EMBRYOLOGY

1 Three week stage: lens placode from surface ectoderm
2 Six week stage: lens vesicle; further development requiring normal neuroretina in appropriate position
3 Twelve week stage: tunica vasculosa lentis
4 Stage at weeks 28–38: degeneration of tunica vasculosa lentis

PHYSIOLOGY

1 Function: refraction of light to produce clear retinal image = 35% of refracting power of eye
2 Growth:
  (a) new fibres formed throughout life
  (b) weight at birth: 100 mg

    (c) weight at 65 years: 250 mg
    (d) width and cell density increase with age
    (e) radius of surface decreases with age
3 Transparency:
    (a) 80% of light between 400 and 1400 nm transmitted
    (b) related to:
        (i) scarcity of cellular organelles
        (ii) little extracellular space
        (iii) high proportion of soluble proteins
    (c) refractive index variable:
        (i) cortex = 1·38
        (ii) nucleus = 1·40
    (d) ageing:
        (i) yellowing of nucleus
        (ii) increased absorption of UV light, aiding retinal protection
        (iii) fluorescent compounds produced (chromatophores)
4 Metabolism:
    (a) anaerobic
    (b) 85% of glucose by glycolysis
    (c) lactate diffuses into aqueous
    (d) 15% by pentose phosphate shunt
    (e) highest metabolic rate in cortex
    (f) energy required for:
        (i) glutathione production
        (ii) large molecule production
        (iii) ion transportation
5 Composition:
    (a) 64% water
    (b) 35% protein (highest in body tissue)
    (c) 1% lipid, trace elements, carbohydrates
    (d) proteins:
        (i) insoluble albuminoid 12%
        (ii) α-crystallins 31%
        (iii) β heavy crystallins ⎱
        (iv) β light crystallins ⎰ 55%
        (v) γ-crystallins 2%
    (e) $[K^+]$ lens: $\times 25$ $[K^+]$ aqueous
    (f) $[Na^+]$ lens: $\times 0·1$ $[Na^+]$ aqueous
    (g) [amino acid] lens: $\times 6$ [amino acid] aqueous
    (h) high glutathione content maintains reduced proteins and membrane pump integrity
6 Accommodation:
    (a) lens essentially non-compressible
    (b) resting state: globular
    (c) relaxed ciliary ring tightens zonules and produces a flattened lens
    (d) ciliary contraction relaxes zonules and results in an increasingly spherical lens; anterior surface shows most increase in curvature (possibly related to differential thickening of anterior capsule)
    (e) ageing:
        (i) less deformable lens

(ii) reduced accommodation

(iii) presbyopia (age 40–45 years)

DISORDERS OF LENS SHAPE AND POSITION

1 Coloboma:
   (a) congenital
   (b) absence of segment of zonule
   (c) lens rim relaxes
   (d) lower quadrants
   (e) associated with iris, choroidal, and optic nerve colobomas, and giant retinal tears
2 Lenticonus:
   (a) conical shape relative to lens surface
   (b) anterior or posterior
   (c) oil drop sign on eliciting red reflex
   (d) irregular myopic lenticular astigmatism
   (e) anterior lenticonus associated with cataract and Alport's syndrome:
       (i) autosomal recessive
       (ii) anterior lenticonus
       (iii) endothelial changes
       (iv) cataract
       (v) spherophakia
       (vi) deafness
       (vii) nephritis
   (f) posterior lenticonus unilateral and associated with cataract prone to rupture on hydrodissection
3 Lentiglobus: generalised hemispherical deformity
4 Microphakia:
   (a) small lens resulting from arrested lens development
   (b) associated with Lowe's syndrome (oculocerebrorenal syndrome)
5 Microspherophakia:
   (a) small spherical lens, usually bilateral
   (b) zonule visible on pupillary dilatation
   (c) iridodonesis
   (d) zonular rupture common
   (e) pupil block glaucoma occurs
   (f) associations:
       (i) familial
       (ii) Weill–Marchesani syndrome
       (iii) Marfan's syndrome
       (iv) hyperlysinaemia
6 Ectopia lentis:
   (a) subluxation or dislocation of lens
   (b) results from zonular rupture
   (c) produces loss of accommodation
   (d) refractive errors may occur:
       (i) subluxation—myopia or astigmatism (lens tilt)
       (ii) dislocation—hypermetropia
   (e) glaucoma caused by lens position or uveitis

Causes of a dislocated lens

1 Hereditary causes:
  (a) Marfan's syndrome
  (b) Weill–Marchesani syndrome
  (c) homocystinuria
  (d) Ehlers–Danlos syndrome
  (e) sulphite oxidase deficiency
  (f) hyperlysinaemia
  (g) familial ectopia lentis (autosomal recessive)
  (h) aniridia
2 Acquired causes:
  (a) trauma: ocular contusion and couching
  (b) buphthalmos
  (c) anterior uveal tumours
  (d) syphilis
  (e) spontaneous (hypermature cataract)
  (f) high myopia
  (g) chronic uveitis

Marfan's syndrome AD   *commonest cause in childhood*
Autosomal dominant; gene defect located on chromosome 15; mesodermal dysplasia; defect of fibrillin synthesis; increased hydroxyproline and desmosine excretion. Clinical diagnosis: arm span > height.
1 General features:
  (a) dissecting aortic aneurysms
  (b) aortic regurgitation
  (c) arachnodactyly; high arched palate
  (d) muscular underdevelopment
2 Ocular features:
  (a) bilateral upward subluxation, *inferior zonules breaks first*
  (b) non-progressive subluxation; accommodation retained *(zonules only elongated not broken)*
  (c) microspherophakia
  (d) angle anomalies (glaucoma)
  (e) hypoplastic iris dilators
  (f) cornea plana — *cloudy*
  (g) axial myopia
  (h) vitreoretinal degeneration and retinal detachment

Weill–Marchesani syndrome
Autosomal recessive; disorder of connective tissue.
1 General features:
  (a) mental handicap
  (b) short stature
  (c) stubby fingers
  (d) joint stiffness
2 Ocular features:
  (a) microphthalmos
  (b) myopia (−10 to −20 D)
  (c) microspherophakia

114

(d) inferior, anterior, or posterior dislocation of lens
(e) glaucoma secondary to lens dislocation

Homocystinuria

Autosomal recessive; deficiency of cystathione synthetase; variable activity produces variable clinical picture; accumulation of methionine and homocystine; nitroprusside urine test and amino acid assays are diagnostic.

1 General features:
  (a) skeletal (osteoporosis, fractures)
  (b) CNS (mental handicap, seizures)
  (c) CVS (malar flush; thromboemboli especially after general anaesthetic)
2 Ocular features:
  (a) acquired zonular damage
  (b) downward subluxation
  (c) staphylomas
  (d) buphthalmos, myopia
  (e) glaucoma; vitreoretinal degeneration ← ophi atrophy.
3 Treatment:
  (a) vitamin B_6 (50% respond)
  (b) methionine restricted diet
  (c) supplementary cystine
  (d) folate

Ehlers–Danlos syndrome AD

Autosomal dominant, autosomal recessive, or X-linked recessive; major defect of type III collagen. At least nine types.

1 General features:
  (a) variable
  (b) hyperextensible joints
  (c) hyperextensible skin
  (d) easy bruising
  (e) poor wound healing
2 Ocular features:
  (a) easy lid eversion (Metenier's sign)
  (b) epicanthic folds
  (c) myopia, microcornea
  (d) blue sclera
  (e) keratoconus
  (f) ectopia lentis
  (g) vitreous haemorrhage
  (h) angioid streaks
  (i) retinal detachment

Sulphite oxidase deficiency

Autosomal recessive; possible deficiency of molybdenum; increased urinary sulphite.

1 General features:
  (a) mental handicap
  (b) frontal bossing

115

2 Ocular features:
   (a) enophthalmos
   (b) ectopia lentis
   (c) Brushfield's spots

Hyperlysinaemia
Autosomal recessive; deficiency of lysine dehydrogenase.
1 General features:
   (a) motor retardation
   (b) mental handicap
   (c) growth retardation
2 Ocular feature: microspherophakia

LENS INDUCED DISORDERS

1 Glaucoma:
   (a) phakomorphic (caused by lens shape/size)
   (b) phakolytic (resulting from capsular leakage/hypermaturity)
   (c) lens displacement
2 Uveitis:
   (a) phakoanaphylactic (autoimmune sensitivity to lens protein)
   (b) phakotoxic (toxic reaction to lens protein)

CATARACT

Definition
Any opacity within the lens; WHO estimates (1978)—15 million blind
(<3/60) from cataract (most common cause of blindness).

Classification

1 According to age:
   (a) congenital
   (b) infantile
   (c) juvenile
   (d) presenile
   (e) senile
2 According to stage:
   (a) immature
   (b) stationary
   (c) progressive
   (d) mature
   (e) intumescent
   (f) hypermature (morgagnian)
3 According to morphology:
   (a) capsular:
        (i) congenital—anterior polar, pyramidal

(ii) acquired—infrared (glassblowers), mercury (grey), chlorpromazine (white star)
(b) subcapsular:
  (i) posterior—senile or secondary, e.g. myotonic dystrophy, corticosteroid induced
  (ii) anterior—*glaukomflecken*, Wilson's disease (green sunflower), miotic therapy
(c) cortical:
  (i) congenital—blue/brown dot; coronary (supranuclear)
  (ii) acquired—senile cuneiform
(d) nuclear:
  (i) congenital—embryonal (cataracta centralis pulverulenta), lamellar with or without riders (genetic, metabolic, and infective causes)
  (ii) acquired—senile nuclear sclerosis
4 According to aetiology:
  (a) not associated with ocular disease
  (b) associated with ocular disease
  (c) associated with systemic disease

Cataracts not associated with ocular disease

Senile cataract; 90% of >70 year age group.
1 Type:
  (a) anterior subcapsular caused by fibrous metaplasia
  (b) posterior subcapsular caused by epithelial cell migration
  (c) cortical
  (d) nuclear cataract is an exaggeration of ageing process
2 Risks:
  (a) increased by:
    (i) smoking
    (ii) dehydration, e.g. diarrhoea
    (iii) UV light exposure
  (b) reduced by non-steroidal anti-inflammatory drugs
3 Lens findings:
  (a) increase in sodium ions, water (hydration), calcium ions, and insoluble proteins
  (b) reduction in potassium ions, amino acids, and glutathione
  (c) changes in crystallins occur caused by deamination, glycosylation, carbamoylation, and sterol addition; these changes result in:
    (i) protein unfolding
    (ii) reduction in thiol groups
    (iii) disulphide cross links
    (iv) changes in surface charges (removal of positive charge)
    (v) exposure of hydrophobic sites
    (vi) protein aggregation
    (vii) increased insoluble protein
    (viii) reduced glutathione levels
4 Lens opacities occur resulting from:
  (a) altered refractive index

(b) large aggregates
(c) differences of refractive index at interfaces

Cataracts associated with ocular disease

1 Congenital disorders:
   (a) aniridia
   (b) hyperplastic primary vitreous
   (c) hereditary retinal disease
   (d) hereditary vitreoretinal disease
2 Acquired disorders:
   (a) uveitis
   (b) glaucoma (*glaukomflecken*)
   (c) myopia
   (d) retinal detachment
   (e) neoplasia
   (f) drug treatment, e.g. steroids, miotics
   (g) trauma:
        (i) contusion (Vossius' lenticular ring)
        (ii) rupture of lens
        (iii) retained intraocular foreign body (siderosis, chalcosis)
        (iv) electric shock
        (v) radiation
        (vi) alkali burns

Cataracts associated with systemic disease

1 Maternal:
   (a) rubella
        (i) 15% of childbearing women susceptible
        (ii) longlasting immunity follows infection
        (iii) fetal risk 80% in first trimester
        (iv) general features:
             • stillbirth or abortion
             • deafness (90%)
             • cardiovascular defects, e.g. patent ductus arteriosus
             • intrauterine growth retardation
             • psychomotor retardation
             • pneumonitis
        (v) ocular features:
             • 30–60%
             • cataract in 50%; unilateral or bilateral; nuclear or diffuse
             • viable virus in lens for 3 years
             • intense uveitis on lens extraction
             • microphthalmos (15%)
             • retinopathy with "salt and pepper" appearance 20 º/º
             • late disciform degeneration, therefore tendency to operate on unilateral cataracts in rubella
             • glaucoma (10%)
             • strabismus, nystagmus, refractive errors, and optic atrophy

    (b) cytomegalovirus inclusion disease:
- (i) general features:
  - low birth weight
  - hepatosplenomegaly, jaundice
  - purpura, pneumonitis
  - cerebral calcification, deafness
  - psychomotor retardation, seizures
- (ii) ocular features:
  - cataract
  - uveitis, microphthalmos
  - optic nerve hypoplasia, coloboma, and atrophy
  - chorioretinitis

    (c) toxoplasmosis: infection of cats and spread via cat faeces; human infection commonly occurs as a result of eating undercooked meat with cysts, e.g. beef and pork:
- (i) general features (nervous system):
  - convulsions
  - mental handicap
  - intracranial calcification
- (ii) ocular features: chorioretinal scars

2 Maternal drug ingestion

3 Maternal radiation

4 Chromosomal abnormalities, e.g. Down's syndrome (snowflake cataract)

5 Hereditary disorders, e.g. Marfan's syndrome and syndromes associated with retinitis pigmentosa

6 Cutaneous disorders:
- (a) atopic dermatitis:
  - (i) anterior or posterior stellate cataract
  - (ii) chronic keratoconjunctivitis
  - (iii) keratoconus
- (b) Werner's syndrome (scleropoikiloderma/progeria)
- (c) Schafer's syndrome (congenital dyskeratoses)
- (d) Rothmund's syndrome (infantile poikiloderma)
- (e) congenital ichthyosis

7 Systemic infections, e.g. syphilis

8 Systemic drugs, e.g. steroids, antimitotics, and chlorpromazine

9 Metabolic disorders:
- (a) diabetes mellitus (bilateral, white snowflake, and may progress rapidly)
- (b) hypoglycaemic cataract
- (c) galactosaemia: autosomal recessive; impairment of galactose metabolism, excess reduced to dulcitol; initially lens clear, osmotic cataract develops; 2 types of defect:
  - (i) galactose-1-phosphate uridyltransferase deficiency with general features:
    - onset in infancy with failure to thrive
    - renal disease
    - hepatosplenomegaly, cirrhosis
    - anaemia, deafness

- mental handicap
- death unless milk and derivatives removed from diet
  - (ii) galactokinase deficiency with general features:
    - systemically well
    - mild galactosaemia possibly associated with presenile cataract
- (d) mannosidosis: α-mannosidase deficiency
  - (i) general features:
    - "Hurler like" syndrome (mental handicap, short stature, skeletal changes, hepatosplenomegaly)
  - (ii) ocular features:
    - posterior spoke like capsular opacity
    - no corneal changes, unlike Hurler's syndrome
- (e) Fabry's disease: α-galactosidase A deficiency:
  - (i) general features:
    - angiokeratomas
    - cardiovascular disorders
    - renal disorders
    - bouts of pain in digits
  - (ii) ocular features:
    - cornea verticillata
    - spoke like cataract (25%)
- (f) Lowe's syndrome: defect of amino acid metabolism:
  - (i) general features:
    - M > F
    - mental handicap
    - renal dwarfism
    - osteomalacia
    - muscular hypotonia
    - frontal prominence
  - (ii) ocular features:
    - congenital glaucoma (50%)
    - congenital cataract (100%)
    - small disc like lens opacities in mother
- (g) Wilson's disease: α_2-globulin (ceruloplasmin) deficiency:
  - (i) general features: hepatolenticular degeneration
  - (ii) ocular features:
    - Kayser–Fleischer ring at level of Descemet's membrane
    - green sunflower cataract
- (h) hypocalcaemia caused by hypoparathyroidism or pseudohypoparathyroidism (short stature and short 4th and 5th metacarpals):
  - (i) ocular features: white dot or coloured crystal opacities
10 Muscular disorders: myotonic dystrophy; autosomal dominant:
  - (a) general features:
    - (i) wasting (temporalis, sternomastoid)
    - (ii) frontal balding
    - (iii) excessive contractility of muscles
    - (iv) hypogonadism
    - (v) cardiac defects
    - (vi) infertility

(b) ocular features:
  (i) ptosis
  (ii) Christmas tree cataract (cortical polychromatic dusting)
  (iii) light/near dissociation
  (iv) pigmentary retinal changes

Assessment of a patient with cataract

1 History: variable and may include:
   (a) changing refraction
   (b) increasing myopia (second sight)
   (c) gradually failing vision
   (d) worse for reading
   (e) worse in bright light
   (f) glare
   (g) ghosting (monocular diplopia)
   (h) monochromatic haloes
   (i) past ocular disease
   (j) past and present refractive status
2 Examination:
   (a) vision (near, distance, and with pinhole)
   (b) refraction
   (c) light projection
   (d) macular function tests
   (e) ocular adnexae
   (f) tears
   (g) cornea (scarring, pannus)
   (h) endothelium (guttata)
   (i) anterior chamber depth
   (j) aqueous inflammation/cells/flare
   (k) intraocular pressure
   (l) pupil:
       (i) afferent defect
       (ii) miosis
       (iii) facility of dilatation
       (iv) synechiae
   (m) cataract morphology and stage
   (n) funduscopy (pre- and postdilatation)
   (o) biometry
3 General:
   (a) age
   (b) occupation
   (c) domestic circumstances
   (d) mental state
   (e) cardiovascular disorders
   (f) respiratory disorders
   (g) prostatic disorders
   (h) metabolic disorders
   (i) drug history
   (j) allergies

Indications for cataract extraction

1 Visual
2 Medical:
  (a) retinal views, e.g. diabetic retinopathy
  (b) lens induced disease
3 Cosmetic

Methods of cataract extraction

1 Intracapsular
2 Extracapsular
3 Lensectomy
4 Lens aspiration
5 Phakoemulsification

Causes of congenital cataracts

1 Idiopathic (largest group)
2 Heredity (25% of congenital cataracts); usually autosomal dominant
3 Maternal infection, e.g. rubella, cytomegalovirus, herpes simplex, *Toxoplasma* sp., varicella-zoster
4 Maternal drug ingestion
5 Maternal malnutrition, e.g. vitamin D deficiency
6 Metabolic disorders, e.g. galactosaemia, hypocalcaemia, amino-aciduria (Lowe's oculocerebrorenal syndrome), hypoglycaemia
7 Chromosomal abnomalities, e.g. Down's syndrome, Turner's syndrome, *cri-du-chat* syndrome
8 Systemic disorders, e.g oxycephaly, Rubinstein–Taybi syndrome
9 Intraocular disease, e.g. uveitis
10 Prematurity

Management of congenital cataract

1 Early detection and treatment important
2 Visual deprivation during sensitive period (first few months of life) results in degeneration of lateral geniculate cells
3 Assessment:
  (a) ocular:
      (i) unilateral means poorer prognosis for vision
      (ii) density of opacity
      (iii) morphology related to aetiology
      (iv) associated ocular pathology
      (v) visual function:
          • history, observation
          • nystagmus (poor prognosis)
          • specific tests, e.g. preferential looking and visual evoked potentials
  (b) general:
      (i) rubella IgM titres
      (ii) viral cultures
      (iii) urine for reducing substances and amino acid assay

      (iv) blood glucose and calcium
      (v) skull radiograph

4 Parents:
   (a) cause of cataract
   (b) motivation for care of child, e.g. contact lens wear

9
RETINAL DETACHMENT AND VITREOUS DISORDERS

Retina

1 Transparent light sensitive membrane
2 Lines inside of eye behind ora serrata
3 Divided into inner neurosensory layer and outer retinal pigment epithelium

Ora serrata

1 Anterior termination of retina
2 Situated 8 mm from nasal limbus
3 Situated 8·5 mm from temporal limbus
4 Thirty five serrations interdigitate with pars plana
5 Firmly adherent to vitreous base
6 Cystic changes occur with age

Bruch's membrane

1 Separates choriocapillaris from retinal pigment epithelium (RPE)
2 Five layers:
    (a) basement membrane of RPE
    (b) inner collagenous layer
    (c) elastic layer
    (d) outer collagenous layer
    (e) basement membrane of choriocapillaris

Retinal pigment epithelium

1 Features:
    (a) single layer hexagonal epithelial cells
    (b) base in contact with Bruch's membrane
    (c) apex in contact with photoreceptors
    (d) contains melanin granules
    (e) apical zona occludens
    (f) at fovea, cells taller and more numerous
    (g) heaped around optic disc
    (h) in periphery larger and irregular

2 Functions:
   (a) maintenance of photoreceptors
   (b) absorption of stray light
   (c) outer blood–retina barrier
   (d) regeneration of visual pigment
   (e) phagocytosis
   (f) active transport of metabolites
3 Age related changes:
   (a) thickening of basement membrane
   (b) drusen formation
   (c) macrophage invasion of drusen
   (d) loss of basal connections
   (e) cellular thinning
   (f) decreased number of nuclei
   (g) pigment clumping
4 Embryology:
   (a) develops from optic cup
   (b) pigmented between 6 and 12 weeks of gestation

Neurosensory retina

1 Layers:
   (a) outer segment of photoreceptor
   (b) outer limiting membrane and cilium of photoreceptor
   (c) outer nuclear layer (8 layers deep); nuclei of photoreceptors
   (d) outer plexiform layers (synapse)
   (e) inner nuclear layer (5 layers deep); nuclei of bipolar cells, horizontal cells, amacrine cells, Müller's cells
   (f) inner plexiform layer (synapse)
   (g) ganglion cell layer
   (h) nerve fibre layer
   (i) inner limiting membrane (Müller's cell end plates)
2 Photoreceptors: light sensitive cells; 2 types: rods and cones
   (a) rods: 120 million; 50 μm long:
      (i) outer segment:
         • modified cilium
         • composed of 1000 stacked discs
         • separate from cell membrane
         • contains visual pigment
         • discs formed at proximal end
         • shed distally in packets
         • rate of shedding 1–5 per hour; increased in light
         • total turnover in 10–14 days
      (ii) cilium—microtubular structure
      (iii) inner segment:
         • outer (ellipsoid) containing mitochondria
         • inner (myoid) containing Golgi bodies and ribosomes
      (iv) outer fibre
      (v) nucleus

(vi) inner fibre
(vii) synaptic region—invaginated area (triad) containing processes from bipolar and horizontal cells
(b) cones: 6 million; 25 μm long; 85 μm long at fovea:
    (i) outer segment:
        • conical
        • stacked saccules (connected to cell membrane)
        • regenerated over 9 months
    (ii) cilium
    (iii) inner segment
    (iv) outer fibre
    (v) nucleus
    (vi) inner fibre—long in foveal cones (Henle's layer)
    (vii) synaptic region—contains 20 triads
3 Modulating cells:
  (a) horizontal cells
  (b) amacrine cells
4 Bipolar cells:
  (a) first order neurons
  (b) connect photoreceptors to ganglion cells
5 Ganglion cells:
  (a) 1000 000 (125 000 from macula)
  (b) second order neurons
  (c) connect bipolar cells to lateral geniculate body cells
  (d) large nuclei, piled 8 deep at macula
  (e) absent at fovea
  (f) all or none response to stimuli
  (g) coded response (opponent cells)
  (h) at fovea: cone:ganglion cell = 1:1
  (i) at periphery: rod:ganglion cell = 10 000:1
6 Müller's cells:
  (a) glial supporting cells
  (b) basement membrane forms inner limiting membrane
  (c) ramify widely down to outer limiting membrane
  (d) functions:
    (i) support
    (ii) nutrition
    (iii) ionic reservoir
    (iv) repair (gliosis)

Embryology of retina

1 Three weeks: optic vesicle formed
2 Six weeks: optic cup formed; initially 10 cells deep:
  (a) outer layer forms retinal pigment epithelium
  (b) inner layer forms sensory retina; differentiation starts at posterior pole
3 Twelve weeks: 2 layered inner retina, separated by transient fibre layer:
  (a) inner neuroblastic layer develops first; forms ganglion, amacrine, and Müller's cells

(b) outer neuroblastic layer invades transient fibre layer; forms horizontal, bipolar, and photoreceptor cells

4 Twenty two weeks: overall adult structure

Photochemistry

1 Visual pigments contained in photoreceptor outer segments
2 Outer segment cell membrane allows entry of sodium ions
3 Inner segment actively secretes sodium producing a current in the resting state (dark current)
4 Light causes changes in the pigment such that calcium ions are released blocking sodium channels, producing a graded hyperpolarisation of the receptor, resulting in reduced neurotransmitter release

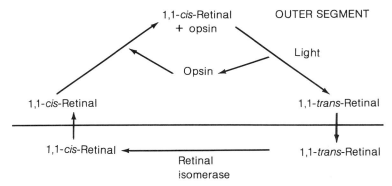

Figure 9.1 The visual cycle

Response to light

1 Rod maximal at 500 nm
2 Red cone maximal at 570 nm
3 Green cone maximal at 535 nm
4 Blue cone maximal at 440 nm

Ocular sensitivity

1 Photopic maximal at 555 nm
2 Scotopic maximal at 507 nm (Purkinje shift)

Dark adaptation

Increasing ocular sensitivity with time in darkness.
1 Initial faster cone adaptation
2 Slower but greater increase in rod sensitivity; maximal at 30–45 min

Retinal image

Transformation of light into membrane potentials; intraretinal processing.

1 Primary image from photoreceptors
2 Secondary image produced in bipolars and modified by horizontal cells
3 Tertiary image produced in ganglion cells and modified by amacrine cells (opponent theory)

Colour vision

Three types of cones responding to primary colours (trichromacy theory); intraretinal processing occurs such that colour is coded along the yellow–blue and red–green axes.

Vitreous

1 Features:
    (a) virtually acellular viscous content of globe
    (b) framework of collagen fibrils reinforced with hyaluronic acid molecules
    (c) 98% water
    (d) volume = 4·5 ml in emmetropic eye
    (e) cortical vitreous contains a higher concentration of collagen fibrils; deficient over premacular and peripapillary areas
    (f) gel vitreous contains membranelles
2 Condensations:
    (a) boundary:
        (i) anterior hyaloid membrane
        (ii) posterior hyaloid membrane
    (b) central: divides gel into tracts
    (c) tubular axial tract (Cloquet's canal)
3 Attachments:
    (a) vitreous base
        (i) 3–4 mm annular attachment
        (ii) very strong
        (iii) extends across ora serrata
    (b) Weigert's ligament: 8–9 mm annular attachment to posterior lens surface (anterior end of Cloquet's canal)
    (c) vitreopapillary adhesions: at posterior end of Cloquet's canal; visible as the Weiss ring following posterior vitreous detachment
    (d) vascular adhesions
    (e) areas of vitreoretinal degenerations, e.g. lattice degeneration, cystic retinal tufts
4 Ageing changes:
    (a) dissociation of hyaluronic acid from fibrils
    (b) pooling of hyaluronic acid
    (c) fibril degeneration and reduced elasticity
    (d) drainage of hyaluronic acid into retrovitreal space (producing posterior vitreous detachment)
5 Function: important in oculogenesis
6 Embryology:
    (a) primary vitreous:
        (i) develops at 5 weeks
        (ii) vascularised

      (iii) attached to optic cup and lens vesicle
- (b) secondary vitreous:
  - (i) complete by 28 weeks
  - (ii) secreted by ciliary body
  - (iii) avascular
- (c) tertiary vitreous:
  - (i) develops at 24 weeks
  - (ii) forms lens zonule

Rhegmatogenous retinal detachment

Retinal detachment occurring in association with retinal hole formation; incidence 1 in 10 000 per year.

1 Predisposing conditions:
  - (a) acute posterior vitreous detachment
  - (b) increasing age
  - (c) myopia (especially high myopia)
  - (d) trauma
  - (e) aphakia (1% after intracapsular extraction, 0·1% after extracapsular extraction with intact posterior capsule)
  - (f) vitreoretinal degenerations
2 Pathogenesis of detachment:
  - (a) dynamic vitreoretinal traction occurs at points of abnormal adhesion following posterior vitreous detachment
  - (b) this results in transmission of energy to retina
  - (c) break formation may relieve traction
  - (d) subretinal fluid may collect causing detachment
  - (e) sensory retina detaches from RPE
  - (f) retina becomes oedematous and opaque
  - (g) photoreceptor degeneration occurs
  - (h) vitreous haemorrhage may result from vascular traction
  - (i) RPE cells may be avulsed into vitreous causing "tobacco dust" and predispose to proliferative vitreoretinopathy
3 Types of break:
  - (a) horseshoe or U shaped tear
  - (b) atrophic hole
4 Causes: myopia; increasing age
  - (a) operculated
  - (b) dialysis:
    - (i) involves splitting of vitreous base
    - (ii) usually inferotemporal
    - (iii) causes: spontaneous; trauma
  - (c) macular hole; causes: idiopathic; commotio retinae; myopia
  - (d) giant retinal tear:
    - (i) 90–360° tears
    - (ii) may fold back
    - (iii) associated with proliferative vitreoretinopathy
    - (iv) causes: trauma; myopia; Stickler's syndrome
  - (e) bucket handle tears:
    - (i) usually superonasal

      (ii) avulsion of vitreous base
      (iii) cause: trauma
  (f) necrotising, e.g. cytomegalovirus retinitis

5 Symptoms:
  (a) photopsia
  (b) floaters
  (c) shadow
  (d) 60% of patients with detachment have all these symptoms

6 Examination:
  (a) visual acuity
  (b) visual fields
  (c) extent of detachment
  (d) distribution and amount of subretinal fluid
  (e) presence of "high water" marks
  (f) position and type of retinal hole using 3-mirror contact lens and indirect ophthalmoscopy with indentation techniques
  (g) presence of vitreoretinal traction
  (h) incidental findings:
      (i) mild anterior uveitis
      (ii) low intraocular pressure
      (iii) tobacco dust in vitreous

7 Natural history:
  (a) progression to total detachment
  (b) spontaneous reattachment (may occur)
  (c) retinal and RPE atrophy
  (d) "high water" mark (reactive hyperplasia of RPE at junction of attached retina)
  (e) viscous subretinal fluid
  (f) intraretinal cyst formation
  (g) proliferative vitreoretinopathy
  (h) rubeosis iridis
  (i) phthisis

8 Treatment principles:
  (a) localisation and closure of breaks
  (b) relief of vitreoretinal traction
      (i) scleral buckling
      (ii) vitrectomy
  (c) production of RPE and neuroretinal adhesion:
      (i) photocoagulation
      (ii) cryotherapy
  (d) internal tamponade:
      (i) air
      (ii) longer acting gases: SF_6, C_3F_8
      (iii) silicone oil
      (iv) heavy liquids (usually intraoperative only)
  (e) treatment of predisposing lesions in fellow eye

9 Complications of cryotherapy:
  (a) proliferative vitreoretinopathy
  (b) uveitis
  (c) pigment granules in vitreous and subretinal space

    (d) cystoid macular oedema
    (e) reactive choroidal hyperaemia
    (f) intraocular haemorrhage
    (g) chorioretinal necrosis
10 Indications for drainage of subretinal fluid:
    (a) large amount of subretinal fluid preventing break localisation
    (b) vitreous traction
    (c) longstanding detachment
    (d) to allow tamponade without occluding the central retinal artery
11 Complications of subretinal fluid drainage:
    (a) haemorrhage
    (b) retinal tear
    (c) retinal incarceration
    (d) hypotony
    (e) vitreous loss
    (f) infection
12 Complications of detachment surgery:
    (a) ischaemia of anterior or posterior segments
    (b) infection
    (c) perforation
    (d) erosion of plomb (external buckling device) into eye
    (e) extrusion of plomb
    (f) muscle imbalance
    (g) changes in refraction
    (h) macular pucker
    (i) cataract
    (j) glaucoma
    (k) redetachment

Proliferative vitreoretinopathy

1 Grade A: pigment clumping in vitreous; pigment cells on retinal surface; vitreous flare
2 Grade B: wrinkling of retina; tears with rolled or irregular edges; vessel tortuosity; decreased vitreous mobility
3 Grade C: full thickness retinal folds—single, multiple, or diffuse; subretinal strands or bands—circumferential contraction produces central displacement; ciliary body and iris traction

Vitreoretinal degenerations

1 Predisposing to retinal detachments:
    (a) lattice degeneration; present in 40% of detached retinae
    (b) snail track degeneration
    (c) white without pressure
2 Benign:
    (a) white with pressure
    (b) pigment clumping
    (c) diffuse chorioretinal atrophy
    (d) peripheral microcystoid changes

    (e) snowflake degeneration
    (f) pavingstone degeneration
    (g) honeycomb degeneration
    (h) drusen
    (i) oral pigmentary degeneration

Causes of traction retinal detachments

1 Penetrating ocular trauma
2 Proliferative retinopathies:
    (a) diabetes mellitus
    (b) sickle cell retinopathy
    (c) retinopathy of prematurity
    (d) retinal vein occlusion
    (e) Eales' disease
3 Persistent hyperplastic primary vitreous
4 Toxocariasis
5 Pars planitis

Causes of exudative retinal detachments

1 Uveitis, e.g. Vogt–Koyanagi–Harada syndrome
2 Choroidal tumour:
    (a) malignant melanoma
    (b) metastatic
3 Glomerulonephritis (hypoproteinaemia)
4 Hypertension
5 Eclampsia
6 Hypothyroidism
7 Choroidal effusion syndrome

Hereditary conditions associated with retinal detachments

1 Marfan's syndrome
2 Wagner's disease
3 Stickler's disease
4 Familial exudative vitreoretinopathy
5 Norrie's disease

Retinoschisis

Splits or cysts within neurosensory retinal layers.
1 Senile: splits in outer plexiform layer:
    (a) features:
        (i) bilateral in 33%
        (ii) usually inferotemporal
        (iii) usually hypermetropic
        (iv) dome elevation of inner retinal layers
        (v) white dots on inner limiting membrane
        (vi) beaten metal appearance of inner leaf
        (vii) sheathing of peripheral retinal vessels
        (viii) round holes can occur in inner leaf

     (ix) larger holes can occur in outer leaf
     (x) 1% progress to rhegmatogenous retinal detachments
     (xi) field defect
  (b) symptoms:
     (i) often none
     (ii) visual field defect if posterior to equator
  (c) management:
     (i) periodic observation, e.g. field charts
     (ii) surgery for subsequent retinal detachment
2 Juvenile: X-linked recessive inheritance; splits in nerve fibre layer; bilateral disorder:
  (a) types:
     (i) foveal
     (ii) peripheral
  (b) associations:
     (i) Goldmann–Favre disease
     (ii) Wagner's disease
  (c) management:
     (i) conservative
     (ii) detachment surgery
     (iii) prognosis poor
3 Secondary:
  (a) causes:
     (i) proliferative retinopathies
     (ii) trauma
     (iii) other causes of vitreous traction
  (b) management: conservative

Vitreous opacities

1 Muscae volitantes: remnants of hyaloid system
2 Syneresis, the Weiss ring (posterior vitreous detachment or PVD), free operculum
3 Haemorrhage
4 Asteroid hyalosis:
  (a) appears in 1 in 200 eyes
  (b) composed of calcium soaps adherent to fibrils
  (c) does not settle at rest
  (d) more common in diabetic people
5 Synchisis scintillans
6 Inflammatory cells:
  (a) pars planitis
  (b) chorioretinitis
7 Neoplastic
8 Amyloid
9 Tobacco dust: pigment cells

Vitreous degenerations

1 Syneresis:
  (a) vitreous liquefaction

   (b) aggregation and condensation of collagen fibrils
   (c) associated with floaters
   (d) causes:
      (i) myopia
      (ii) senescence
      (iii) trauma
      (iv) inflammations
      (v) hereditary: Wagner's disease, Jensen's disease, Stickler's disease

2 Detachment:
   (a) collapse of vitreous gel
   (b) associated with floaters and photopsia
   (c) causes:
      (i) senile
      (ii) myopic
      (iii) postinflammatory
      (iv) postvitreous haemorrhage
      (v) diabetic retinopathy
   (d) PVD with collapsed gel, i.e. total:
      (i) without vitreous haemorrhage—4% develop retinal breaks
      (ii) with vitreous haemorrhage—20% develop breaks
   (e) PVD without collapse, i.e. subtotal
      (i) associated with future retinal hole or vitreous haemorrhage
      (ii) scaffold for new vessels in proliferative retinopathy

Vitreous haemorrhage

1 Causes:
   (a) proliferative retinopathies:
      (i) diabetes mellitus
      (ii) retinal vein occlusion
      (iii) sickle cell retinopathy
      (iv) Eales' disease
      (v) retinopathy of prematurity
   (b) posterior vitreous detachment
   (c) trauma
   (d) disciform macular degeneration
   (e) blood dyscrasias
   (f) subarachnoid haemorrhage (Terson's syndrome)

2 Complications:
   (a) syneresis
   (b) inflammation and fibrosis: leads to traction detachment
   (c) haemosiderosis
   (d) glaucoma, haemolytic, or ghost cell
   (e) synchisis scintillans: cholesterol crystals; settles inferiorly at rest
   (f) ochre membrane

Persistent hyperplastic primary vitreous (PHPV)

1 Anterior (90%):
   (a) unilateral retrolental mass

    (b) elongated ciliary processes
    (c) microphthalmos
    (d) cataract
    (e) secondary angle closure glaucoma
    (f) vitreous haemorrhage
2 Posterior (10%):
    (a) white membrane from optic disc to peripheral retina; usually inferior
    (b) tractional retinal detachment
    (c) "morning glory" syndrome may be a variant

Causes of leukocoria (white pupil, cat's eye pupil)

1 Cataract
2 Retrolental masses:
    (a) persistent hyperplastic primary vitreous
    (b) retinopathy of prematurity
    (c) Norrie's disease
3 Tumours:
    (a) retinoblastoma
    (b) choroidal metastases
4 Exudates:
    (a) familial exudative vitreoretinopathy
    (b) Coats' disease
5 Change in retina or choroid:
    (a) incontinentia pigmenti
    (b) high myopia
    (c) myelinated nerve fibres (extensive)
    (d) retinal dysplasia
    (e) choroidaemia
6 Infections:
    (a) toxocariasis
    (b) endophthalmitis

Indications for vitrectomy

1 Anterior segment conditions:
    (a) accidental vitreous loss during surgery
    (b) lensectomy, e.g. for secondary cataract in childhood arthritis
    (c) excision of pupillary membranes
    (d) vitreous touch causing bullous keratopathy
    (e) incarceration of vitreous in cataract section
    (f) malignant (ciliary block) glaucoma
    (g) glaucoma drainage surgery in aphakic-eyes
2 Posterior segment conditions:
    (a) diabetic disease:
        (i) markedly reduced visual acuity secondary to vitreous haemorrhage
        (ii) tractional retinal detachment involving macula
        (iii) proliferative vitreoretinopathy with macular traction
        (iv) rubeosis with poor retinal view

135

(b) proliferative diseases causing vitreous opacification:
- (i) branch retinal vein occlusion
- (ii) sickle cell disease
- (iii) inflammatory disease
- (iv) Eales' disease

(c) trauma:
- (i) blunt—dislocated lens, vitreous haemorrhage, giant tears
- (ii) foreign body retrieval

(d) complicated retinal detachment, e.g. giant tears, multiple posterior or large retinal breaks, proliferative vitreoretinopathy

(e) interface maculopathy (pucker)

(f) endophthalmitis

(g) vitreous biopsy, removal of persistent opacity, e.g. amyloid

(h) subretinal neovascular membrane removal (younger patients, e.g. in presumed ocular histoplasmosis syndrome)

(i) Idiopathic macular holes

Macular holes

1 Aetiology
- (a) idiopathic
- (b) trauma
- (c) macular disease e.g. diabetic maculopathy

2 Idiopathic macular holes
- (a) commonly perimenopausal women
- (b) 10–20% bilateral
- (c)
  - (i) stage I—loss of foveal reflex, yellow-white spot
  - (i) stage II—irregular, full thickness dehiscence at fovea
  - (i) stage III—round, full thickness hole with overlying operculum
- (d) treatment—vitrectomy and gas

10
RETINAL VASCULAR DISORDERS

BLOOD SUPPLY TO RETINA

1 Central retinal artery:
  (a) first branch of ophthalmic artery
  (b) true artery
  (c) end artery
  (d) divides into upper and lower trunks, usually at optic disc
  (e) accompanied by vein
2 Retinal arteries:
  (a) subdivisions of trunks
  (b) 2 superior and 2 inferior
  (c) histologically: arterioles with little elastic tissue
  (d) surrounded by capillary free zone (120 μm)
3 Cilioretinal artery:
  (a) present in 20% of patients
  (b) supply from posterior ciliary circulation
  (c) supplies variable area of retina
4 Capillaries:
  (a) lined by non-fenestrated endothelium
  (b) capillary walls contain pericytes
  (c) 2 plexus:
      (i) deep
      (ii) superficial
  (d) absent from foveal avascular zones
5 Retinal veins:
  (a) main branches mirror arterioles
  (b) drain to central retinal vein
  (c) share common sheath at arteriovenous crossings
  (d) normal artery:vein ratio 2:3
6 Vascular anomalies:
  (a) divisions into main arterioles may occur on disc or a little way into the retina

(b) anomalous trifurcations associated with disc drusen
(c) congenital tortuosity

PHYSIOLOGY

1 Central retinal artery:
   (a) mean arterial pressure = 75 mm Hg
   (b) arterial pulsations occur if blood pressure < intraocular pressure
   (c) venous pulsation can be seen under normal circumstances
2 Capillaries:
   (a) pressure = 55 mm Hg
   (b) retinal artery–capillary pressure drop caused by increased surface area
   (c) absent precapillary sphincters
   (d) all capillary beds perfused
   (e) capillary endothelial tight junctions account for blood–retina barrier
   (f) capillaries impermeable to proteins, ensuring little extracellular fluid of low osmotic pressure
3 Central retinal vein:
   (a) pressure = 25 mm Hg
4 Retinal perfusion—relates to:
   (a) vascular pressure head
   (b) vascular resistance
   (c) blood viscosity
5 Autoregulation of retinal flow:
   (a) ensures adequate perfusion over range of intraocular pressures
   (b) no neurogenic control
   (c) some chemical control (high Po_2 producing constriction; high Pco_2 producing dilatation)

EMBRYOLOGY

1 Retina initially avascular
2 Retinal arterioles develop as branches of hyaloid artery
3 Extend to equator by 8 months
4 Temporal retina may not be vascularised at birth
5 Capillaries penetrate to inner nuclear layer
6 Central retinal vein develops by 3 months
7 Vascular pattern not genetically determined

DIABETES MELLITUS

1 Disorder of glucose metabolism resulting from diminished availability or effectiveness of insulin
2 Results in an increase in blood glucose concentration
3 Random blood glucose >11·0 mmol/l or fasting blood glucose >8 mmol/l

4 In the UK, 1–2% of the population; 500 000 cases diagnosed and possibly 500 000 undiagnosed

Types

1 Juvenile onset, insulin dependent diabetes (type I):
   (a) often presents acutely with systemic disease: fatigue, weight loss, polyuria, polydipsia, infection, and coma
   (b) multifactorial aetiology:
       (i) viruses (especially Coxsackie B4)
       (ii) genetic predisposition (associated with HLA-DR3, -DR4, -B8, and -B15)
       (iii) pancreatic islet cell antibodies
   (c) peak incidence 11–14 years of age
2 Maturity onset, non-insulin dependent (type II):
   (a) tends to occur in elderly and overweight people
   (b) often asymptomatic
   (c) probably inherited; nearly all identical twins with type II diabetes mellitus have a similarly affected co-twin
   (d) occurs most frequently between the ages of 50 and 70 years
3 Secondary:
   (a) drug induced:
       (i) steroids
       (ii) thiazide diuretics
   (b) endocrine:
       (i) acromegaly
       (ii) Cushing's disease
       (iii) thyrotoxicosis
   (c) pancreatic, e.g. pancreatitis

Features

1 Vascular:
   (a) large vessel disease, e.g. myocardial infarction
   (b) small vessel disease, e.g. renal failure
2 Renal:
   (a) diffuse glomerulosclerosis and nodular glomerulosclerosis (Kimmelstiel–Wilson lesion)
   (b) pyelonephritis and renal capillary necrosis
3 Neuromuscular: mononeuritis, peripheral neuropathy, autonomic neuropathy, and amyotrophy (painful, asymmetrical weakness, and wasting of quadriceps)
4 Skin:
   (a) sensitivity and lipoatrophy at injection sites
   (b) necrobiosis lipoidica diabeticorum over shins
5 Infections, e.g. candidiasis and tuberculosis
6 Ocular:
   (a) blepharitis, styes
   (b) recurrent corneal erosions (corneal hypoanaesthesia)
   (c) iris:
       (i) neuropathy (poor dilatation)

      (ii) pigment loss
      (iii) neovascularisation and secondary glaucoma
  (d) primary open angle glaucoma
  (e) cataracts
  (f) refractive changes in lens (hypermetropia > myopia)
  (g) retinopathy and vitreous haemorrhage
  (h) vitreous haemorrhage
  (i) ischaemic optic neuropathy
  (j) cranial nerve palsies, e.g. nerve III

DIABETIC RETINOPATHY

1 Prevalence of retinopathy at time of diagnosis: 1·5% age 20–40 years; 7% age 50–60 years; 10% in older patients
2 Retinopathy at diagnosis is probably the result of a long period of undiagnosed and often asymptomatic hyperglycaemia in middle aged and elderly diabetic patients
3 Prevalence of retinopathy rises with duration of disease to a peak of 79% 20 years after diagnosis
4 Diabetic retinopathy is the second most common cause of blind and partial sight registration in the 30–60 year age group
5 Fifty per cent of blind diabetic people are dead within 3–4 years of registration and only 20% survive for 10 years

Possible factors in the pathogenesis of diabetic retinopathy

1 Thickening of basement membrane with deposits of glycogen and carbohydrate
2 Capillary endothelial cell damage
3 Biochemical changes in red blood cells leading to defective oxygen transport
4 Increased stickiness and aggregation of platelets
5 Loss of vascular pericytes

Classification

1 Background
2 Maculopathy:
  (a) exudative
  (b) oedematous
  (c) ischaemic
  (d) mixed
3 Pre-proliferative
4 Proliferative
5 Advanced diabetic eye disease:
  (a) persistent vitreous haemorrhage
  (b) retinal detachment
  (c) opaque membrane formation
  (d) neovascular glaucoma

Signs of background diabetic retinopathy

1 Microaneurysms:
   (a) first clinically detectable changes of diabetic retinopathy
   (b) inner nuclear layer of the retina
2 Hard exudates: outer plexiform and inner nuclear layers
3 Haemorrhages:
   (a) flame shaped: retinal nerve fibre layer
   (b) dot and blot: middle retinal layers

Diabetic maculopathy

1 Retinopathy in the macular area
2 Most common cause of visual loss in patients with diabetes mellitus
3 More common in type II diabetic patients

Classification of maculopathy

1 Exudative:
   (a) features:
       (i) exudates in the macular area
       (ii) circinate rings
   (b) management:
       (i) photocoagulation may be beneficial when vision is better than 6/60
       (ii) treatment to centre of circinate rings or sites of leakage
2 Oedematous:
   (a) features:
       (i) macular oedema
       (ii) extracellular fluid in Henle's layer; may be seen by microscopic examination of the macular area or on fluorescein angiography
   (b) management:
       (i) macular grid with low intensity, short duration laser
       (ii) laser before vision worse than 6/18
3 Ischaemic:
   (a) features: fluorescein angiogram reveals capillary non-perfusion
   (b) management:
       (i) no proven treatment
       (ii) 30% proceed to proliferative diabetic retinopathy within 2 years, so may eventually require panretinal photocoagulation
4 Mixed:
   (a) features:
       (i) exudates
       (ii) ischaemia
       (iii) oedema
   (b) management: photocoagulation may be of benefit
5 Indications for macular laser treatment: Early Treatment Diabetic Retinopathy Study (ETDRS); clinically significant macular oedema:
   (a) thickening of the retina at or within 500 μm of the centre of the macula
   (b) exudates at or within 500 μm of the centre of the macula, if

associated with thickening of the adjacent retina
(c) a zone or zones of retinal thickening 1 disc area or larger, any part of which is within 1 disc diameter of the centre of the macula (macular laser halves the rate of severe visual loss in such eyes)

Pre-proliferative diabetic retinopathy

1 Features:
(a) cotton wool spots
(b) venous changes: dilatation and beading of the vessels
(c) arteriolar narrowing
(d) large blotch haemorrhages
(e) intraretinal microvascular abnormalities (IRMAs)
(f) capillary closure on fluorescein angiogram
2 Retinal signs associated with increased risk of progression to proliferative retinopathy (ETDRS report 12):

Table 10.1

Retinal sign	Increased risk with increased severity
Venous beading—single best predictor	Fourfold or more
Haemorrhages/microaneurysms	Fourfold
Intraretinal microvascular abnormalities	Fourfold
Cotton wool spots	Twice

3 Management: photocoagulation (but controversial); some would improve contact and treat only if new vessels develop

Proliferative diabetic retinopathy

1 Incidence:
(a) overall incidence of proliferative change: 10–20%
(b) incidence greater for insulin dependent than for non-insulin dependent diabetic person
2 Pathogenesis:
(a) extensive retinal capillary closure
(b) angiogenesis factor release stimulates proliferation
(c) endothelial buds from the venous end of capillaries, usually at junction of perfused/non-perfused areas
(d) fibrovascular network adherent to vitreous face
(e) vitreous detachment may elevate vessels
(f) new vessels bleed, resulting in further vitreous contraction and retinal detachment
3 Features:
(a) neovascularisation: this is pathognomonic of proliferative diabetic retinopathy; it occurs at the disc (NVD) or elsewhere (NVE)
(b) fibrovascular epiretinal membrane: initially transparent but becomes opaque
(c) vitreous traction with retinal detachment
4 Prognosis (Table 10.2)

Table 10.2

	If untreated risk of severe visual loss in 2 years (%)	If treated with photocoagulation risk of severe visual loss in 2 years (%)
Severe NVD and vitreous haemorrhage	40	20
Moderate to severe NVD, no vitreous haemorrhage	25	5
NVE and vitreous haemorrhage	30	7
NVE, no vitreous haemorrhage	7	7

5 Management:
  (a) photocoagulation
  (b) ensure good control of blood glucose levels; retinopathy may worsen temporarily if control suddenly improves
  (c) stop smoking
  (d) treat systemic hypertension
  (e) avoid heavy physical exertion or strain
  (f) avoid rapid changes in blood glucose levels
  (g) avoid direct trauma
  (h) reduce heavy alcohol consumption

Photocoagulation in proliferative diabetic retinopathy

1 Indications for panretinal photocoagulation in proliferative diabetic retinopathy: Diabetic Retinopathy Study; high risk characteristics:
  (a) optic disc neovascularisation (NVD) of moderate to severe degree
  (b) optic disc neovascularisation (NVD) of any degree if associated with vitreous or preretinal haemorrhage
  (c) retinal neovascularisation (NVE) if associated with vitreous or preretinal haemorrhage
      (panretinal photocoagulation halves the rate of severe visual loss in such eyes)
2 Technique:
  (a) contact lenses: fundus contact lens for macular view, 3 mirror contact lens for peripheral photocoagulation; panfunduscopic lens gives a wider field of vision but inverted image like indirect ophthalmoscope
  (b) mild flat NVE: blanch retinal pigment epithelium; 200–500 μm spot size; 0·02–0·20 second; treat sector and directly
  (c) elevated NVE: as above; direct treatment usually unsuccessful as vessels reopen or bleeding occurs
  (d) moderate to severe NVE: panretinal photocoagulation with 2000–3500 burns; 200–500 μm spot size; 0·02–0·20 second
  (e) NVD: panretinal photocoagulation

Advanced diabetic eye disease

1 Clinical features:
  (a) persistent vitreous haemorrhage

143

   (b) tractional retinal detachment; types of traction:
      (i) tangential
      (ii) anteroposterior
      (iii) bridging traction
   (c) opaque membrane on posterior hyaloid face
   (d) neovascular glaucoma with rubeosis iridis
2 Management:
   (a) vitrectomy
   (b) cutting of traction membranes
   (c) epiretinal membrane peeling
   (d) endolaser
   (e) atropine, steroids, and eventually retrobulbar alcohol and enuclea-
      tion for a painful blind eye
3 Indications for vitrectomy:
   (a) non-clearing vitreous haemorrhage
   (b) macular tractional retinal detachment
   (c) active advanced proliferative retinopathy
   (d) tractional rhegmatogenous retinal detachment
   (e) premacular haemorrhage

HYPERTENSION

1 Definitions (WHO):

(a)	normotension	systolic	<140 mm Hg
		diastolic	<90 mm Hg
(b)	borderline	systolic	>140 to <160 mm Hg
		diastolic	>90 to <95 mm Hg
(c)	hypertension	systolic	>160 mm Hg
		diastolic	>95 mm Hg

2 Causes:
   (a) essential (95%)
   (b) renal disease
   (c) endocrine disease, e.g. Cushing's syndrome, Conn's syndrome,
      phaeochromocytoma, acromegaly
   (d) contraceptive pill and eclampsia
   (e) coarctation of the aorta
3 Histopathology:
   (a) "benign" hypertension:
      (i) arteriole hyalinisation—deposits of eosinophilic material under
         endothelium and eventually in vessel wall
      (ii) small/medium sized arteries—medial muscular hypertrophy
         and fibrosis with intimal proliferation; microaneurysm forma-
         tion in small perforating arteries of the brain
      (iii) large arteries—accelerated atherosclerosis
   (b) "malignant" or accelerated hypertension:
      (i) arterioles—endothelial damage allowing red blood cells and
         plasma to leak into vessel wall where fibrin precipitates = "fib-
         rinoid necrosis" of the arteriolar wall; focal spasm and
         segmental dilatation
4 Complications:
   (a) left ventricular failure

   (b) renal failure
   (c) strokes and hypertensive encephalopathy
   (d) myocardial infarction
   (e) complications of treatment
   (f) retinopathy
5 Ocular features:
   (a) vasoconstriction with arteriolar narrowing (focal)
   (b) leakage leading to haemorrhages, retinal oedema, and exudates
   (c) exudates may deposit radially around the fovea in Henle's layer (macular star)
   (d) cotton wool spots
6 Grading of hypertensive retinopathy:
   (a) grade 1: silver wiring
   (b) grade 2: arteriovenous nipping
   (c) grade 3: grade 2 and haemorrhages, exudates, and cotton wool spots
   (d) grade 4: changes of grade 3 and disc swelling; the general prognosis is the same with grade 3 or grade 4 changes

Signs of arteriosclerotic retinopathy

Usually associated with hypertension.
1 Arteriovenous nipping (Salus' sign)
2 Dilated vein distal to arteriovenous crossing (Bonnet's sign)
3 Tapering of vein on either side of crossing (Gunn's sign)
4 Right angle deflection of vein
5 Silver wiring of arterioles
6 Ischaemic choroidal infarcts (Elschnig's bodies)
7 Retinal arterial macroaneurysm
8 Ischaemic optic neuropathy

Macular star

Star shaped exudates in Henle's layer of the macula; causes:
1 Hypertension
2 Papilloedema
3 Papillitis
4 Ocular or cerebral trauma
5 Obstruction of arteries or veins supplying macular area
6 Retinal periphlebitis
7 Juxtapapillary choroiditis
8 Chronic infections, e.g. tuberculosis, syphilis
9 Idiopathic

Cotton wool spots

1 White fluffy retinal lesions
2 Represent areas of retinal ischaemia which cause disruption of axonal transport
3 Axonal swelling and rupture
4 Products of axonal transport accumulate at end of axon resulting in

"cytoid bodies"

Causes
1 Malignant hypertension
2 Diabetic retinopathy
3 Anaemia
4 Infective conditions, e.g. septicaemia, subacute bacterial endocarditis, acquired immune deficiency syndrome
5 Collagen vascular diseases, e.g. lupus erythematosus, polyarteritis nodosa
6 Retinopathy following crush injuries (Purtscher's disease or angiopathic retinopathy)

Retinal macroaneurysm

1 Features:
  (a) occurs in elderly hypertensive or arteriosclerotic individuals
  (b) single or multiple
  (c) usually at posterior pole
  (d) may:
    (i) occlude spontaneously
    (ii) bleed—pathognomonic feature = trilayer haemorrhage, i.e. sub-retinal, intraretinal, and preretinal haemorrhage
    (iii) leak:
      • circinate exudate
      • macular oedema
2 Management:
  (a) conservative (focal grid)
  (b) photocoagulation if leaking

RETINAL VEIN OCCLUSION

1 Causes:
  (a) pressure on the vein:
    (i) systemic hypertension with arterial pressure on vein (artery and vein share common fibrous sheath)
    (ii) raised intraocular pressure
  (b) vessel wall disease:
    (i) diabetes
    (ii) vessel wall inflammation, e.g. sarcoidosis and Behçet's disease
  (c) increased blood viscosity:
    (i) polycythaemia
    (ii) leukaemia
    (iii) myeloma
    (iv) hyperlipidaemia
2 Clinical features:
  (a) dilated veins
  (b) flame shaped haemorrhages
  (c) retinal oedema
  (d) cotton wool spots

    (e) venous and occasionally arterial sheathing
    (f) exudates
3 Complications:
    (a) macular oedema
    (b) new vessel formation on the optic disc, retina, and also the iris causing secondary glaucoma (hundred day glaucoma)
    (c) neovascularisation may lead to vitreous haemorrhage and tractional retinal detachment
4 Management:
    (a) exclude underlying cause
    (b) photocoagulation if marked ischaemia or neovascularisation is present
    (c) drugs that inhibit coagulation (unproven)

Causes of dilated retinal veins

1 Congenital, e.g. von Hippel–Lindau disease, Wyburn–Mason syndrome
2 Trauma and inflammation, e.g. caroticocavernous fistula, periphlebitis, anterior uveitis, impending obstruction of the central retinal vein
3 Cardiovascular disease
4 Respiratory disease
5 Central nervous system disease, e.g. papilloedema, subarachnoid haemorrhage
6 Haematological diseases, e.g. polycythaemia, leukaemia, myeloma
7 Febrile illnesses, e.g. septicaemia
8 Metabolic diseases, e.g. diabetic retinopathy
9 Collagen vascular diseases, e.g. polyarteritis nodosa
10 Toxic conditions, e.g. methyl alcohol ingestion

Causes of retinal vascular tortuosity

1 Normal variation
2 Congenital
3 Haematological disorders, e.g. polycythaemia, myeloma, cryoglobulinaemia, and sickle cell disease
4 Hypertension
5 Haemangioma of retina
6 Hereditary haemorrhagic telangiectasia
7 Eales' disease
8 Fabry's disease
9 Coats' disease
10 Chronic open angle glaucoma

Causes of juxtafoveolar retinal telangiectasia

1 Small branch vein occlusion
2 Diabetes mellitus
3 Radiotherapy
4 Carotid artery obstruction

5 Hereditary haemorrhagic telangiectasia (Osler–Weber–Rendu syndrome)
6 Fevers
7 Cardiovascular shock
8 Anticoagulant drug therapy
9 Intracranial haemorrhage
10 Haematological disorders
11 Trauma
12 Valsalva haemorrhagic retinopathy
13 Idiopathic

RETINAL ARTERY OCCLUSION

1 Causes:
  (a) external pressure, e.g. raised intraocular pressure, from acute closed angle glaucoma or retinal detachment surgery
  (b) vessel wall occlusion:
    (i) atheroma
    (ii) arteritis, e.g. giant cell arteritis, polyarteritis nodosa, systemic lupus erythematosus
  (c) embolisation:
    (i) carotid (usually occurs at bifurcation)
    (ii) valve problems, e.g. subacute bacterial endocarditis or stenotic lesions
    (iii) cardiac wall problems, e.g. mural thrombus from myocardial infarction, atrial myxoma
2 Types of embolus:
  (a) cholesterol (Hollenhorst's plaques): atheromatous plaques appear as refractile crystals
  (b) fibrinoplatelet: cause amaurosis fugax
  (c) calcific: may cause permanent occlusion of vessel
3 Clinical features:
  (a) sudden loss of vision
  (b) painless
  (c) field defect if branch occlusion
  (d) afferent pupillary defect
  (e) onset after a few hours
  (f) white and oedematous retina with reflex from choroidal vessels showing through at fovea (cherry-red spot); disappears after a few weeks
  (g) up to 18% develop new vessels on the iris (rubeosis iridis)
  (h) optic atrophy with no other features
4 Management:
  (a) acute:
    (i) ocular massage
    (ii) intravenous acetazolamide
    (iii) anterior chamber paracentesis
    (iv) inhalation of high oxygen/high carbon dioxide mixture
    (v) supine position
  (b) exclude underlying causes particularly giant cell arteritis

Causes of a cherry-red spot

1 Central retinal artery occlusion
2 Sphingolipidoses, e.g. Tay–Sachs, Niemann–Pick, Gaucher's diseases
3 Quinine toxicity
4 Traumatic retinal oedema
5 Macular retinal hole with surrounding detachment

SICKLE CELL DISEASE

Sickle cell disease is caused by the presence of one or more abnormal haemoglobins causing blood cells to adopt an abnormal shape under conditions of low oxygen and acidosis. These deformed red blood cells cause a change in blood flow and cause hypoxia.

1 Types:
   (a) AS (sickle cell trait): requires hypoxia or abnormal conditions to produce sickling; mild form
   (b) SS (sickle cell disease): severe systemic complications, mild ocular disease
   (c) SC (sickle cell haemoglobin C disease): severe ocular disease
   (d) S Thal (sickle cell haemoglobin with thalassaemia): severe systemic and ocular disease
2 General features:
   (a) painful crises: caused by tissue infarction; precipitated by infection, dehydration, and low temperature
   (b) aplastic crises: falling haemoglobin level caused by parvovirus B19 infection
   (c) sequestration crises: pooling of sickled erythrocytes in spleen, liver, or lungs
   (d) infection: particularly pneumococcal; also salmonella osteomyelitis
   (e) renal damage
   (f) chronic leg ulceration
   (g) aseptic bone necrosis
3 Ocular features:
   (a) conjunctiva: dark red vascular segments shaped like commas or corkscrews; involves small calibre vessels
   (b) iris:
       (i) focal ischaemic atrophy
       (ii) rubeosis (rare)
       (iii) hyphaema
   (c) retina/choroid:
       (i) venous tortuosity
       (ii) black sun-bursts (peripheral choroidoretinal scars)
       (iii) salmon patch haemorrhages (peripheral pink superficial haemorrhages)
       (iv) refractile spots
       (v) silver wiring of peripheral arterioles
       (vi) retinal breaks *equator + preequator*
       (vii) angioid streaks

149

(viii) vascular occlusions:
- central retinal artery
- macular artery
- retinal vein
- choroid ulcers

(ix) retinopathy

4 Stages of proliferative sickle retinopathy:
  (a) stage 1: peripheral arterial occlusions
  (b) stage 2: peripheral arterioanastomoses (dilated pre-existent capillary channel)
  (c) stage 3: new vesseis from anastomoses (sea-fan neovascularisation)
  (d) stage 4: vitreous haemorrhage
  (e) stage 5: vitreous traction and retinal detachment

5 Management of sickle cell retinopathy:
  (a) photocoagulation
  (b) vitrectomy (late stage of proliferative disease)
  (c) retinal detachment surgery; may be complicated by anterior segment ischaemia and may require exchange transfusion

Causes of retinal fan shaped neovascularisation ("sea-fan")

1 Haemoglobinopathy
2 Retinopathy of prematurity (retrolental fibroplasia)
3 Diabetes mellitus
4 Eales' disease
5 Sarcoidosis
6 Central and branch retinal vein occlusion
7 Uveitis
8 Familial exudative vitreoretinopathy

RETINOPATHY OF PREMATURITY (RETROLENTAL FIBROPLASIA)

1 Definition: a proliferative retinopathy affecting pre-term infants and low weight infants ($<32/40$, <1500 g); sometimes in association with exposure to high ambient oxygen concentrations

2 Classification of cicatricial ROP:
  (a) stage 1: mild peripheral retinal changes including retinal pigmentation and vitreous opacification; myopia common
  (b) stage 2: temporal vitreoretinal traction with dragging of posterior retina
  (c) stage 3: peripheral fibrosis with falciform folds
  (d) stage 4: partial tractional retinal detachment
  (e) stage 5: total retinal detachment; secondary angle closure glaucoma

3 Classification of proliferative ROP:
  (a) location 1:
    (i) zone 1—posterior retina, 60° circle around the optic disc
    (ii) zone 2—from zone 1 to nasal ora serrata
    (iii) zone 3—from zone 3 outward to temporal ova serrata

    (b) extent: described by number of clock hours involved
    (c) severity:
        (i) stage 1—demarcation line between vascularised and non-vascularised retina
        (ii) stage 2—elevation or ridge at demarcation line
        (iii) stage 3—extraretinal fibrovascular proliferation or ridge
        (iv) stage 4—retinal detachment
    (d) "plus" disease:
        (i) dilatation of retinal vessels
        (ii) vitreous haze
        (iii) poor pupillary dilatation
4 Management:
    (a) monitor arterial oxygen (but may develop without exposure to high O_2 levels)
    (b) screen all neonates < 32 weeks or < 1500 g
    (c) treat all stage 3 plus involving > 5 contiguous or 8 accumulative clock hours; cryotherapy or indirect laser
    (d) vitamin E (controversial)
    (e) scleral buckling for detachment (very poor prognosis)

EALES' DISEASE

Retinal periphlebitis of unknown aetiology. Affects young men; bilateral.
1 Clinical features:
    (a) recurrent vitreous haemorrhages
    (b) rubeosis iridis
    (c) neovascular glaucoma
    (d) cataract
2 Stages:
    (a) stage 1: sheathing of retinal venules by inflammatory deposits, retinal oedema, and small retinal haemorrhages
    (b) stage 2: more severe involvement extending into posterior pole with vitreous haze
    (c) stage 3: peripheral retinal neovascularisation
    (d) stage 4: proliferative retinopathy with retinal and vitreous haemorrhage, and tractional retinal detachment
4 Management:
    (a) destroy new vessels and areas of retinal ischaemia
    (b) vitrectomy in certain cases

COATS' DISEASE

1 Clinical features: *in Children. DD - leukocoria -*
                                         DD. Retinoblastoma
    (a) unilateral
    (b) males in first decade
    (c) peripheral telangiectatic and aneurysmal lesions
    (d) massive subretinal exudation resulting in:
        (i) cataract
        (ii) glaucoma
        (iii) retinal detachment

2 Management:
  (a) photocoagulation
  (b) cryotherapy
  (c) retinal detachment surgery

11
MACULA

Macular anatomy

1 Horizontally oval, 5 mm in diameter
2 Centre 4 mm temporal, 0·8 mm inferior to disc
3 Contains more than one ganglion cell layer
4 Xanthophyll pigment in inner retinal layers
5 Specialised areas:
  (a) fovea:
        (i) 1·5 mm diameter (5′ of arc)
       (ii) 6–8 ganglion cell layers
      (iii) thickened internal limiting membrane
      (iv) retinal pigment epithelial (RPE) cells taller, more numerous, and contain more melanosomes
  (b) foveola:
        (i) 0·26 mm diameter (54″ of arc)
       (ii) thinnest part of retina
      (iii) central umbo responsible for foveolar reflection
      (iv) contains only cones (150 000/mm^2)
       (v) cones taller and thinner than elsewhere
      (vi) inner retinal elements displaced laterally
     (vii) cone inner fibres run parallel to retinal surface in Henle's layer with relatively little supporting structure
    (viii) thinned internal limiting membrane
  (c) foveal avascular zone:
        (i) 0·5 mm diameter
       (ii) surrounded by continuous capillary network
      (iii) extent visible only on fluorescein angiography

Symptoms of macular disease

1 Poor vision (especially reading)
2 Central scotoma
3 Hypermetropia (+ 1·0 D lens test)
4 Metamorphopsia

5 Micropsia and macropsia
6 Colour vision defects (red–green)

Examination of a patient with macular disease

1 Vision (near and distance)
2 Colour vision, e.g. colour desaturation
3 Photostress test
4 Amsler grid
5 Maddox rod
6 Perimetry
7 Fundal examination (Hruby, contact lens, +90, +78 D lens)
8 Fluorescein angiography
9 Entoptic phenomena, e.g. flying corpuscle
10 Contrast sensitivity
11 Flicker fusion frequency
12 Electrophysiological tests

Fluorescein angiography

1 Principles:
    (a) excitation of fluorescein at 490 nm (blue)
    (b) fluorescent emission at 530 nm (green)
    (c) fluorescein remains intravascular within the retina, but leaks from the choroidal circulation
    (d) 70–80% of fluorescein protein bound
    (e) 20–30% free fluorescein
2 Technique:
    (a) 5 ml of 10% fluorescein injected intravenously
    (b) 3 ml of 25% fluorescein if media hazy
    (c) arm to eye time about 9 seconds
3 Phases:
    (a) prearterial: choroidal flush
    (b) arterial: 1 second later
    (c) capillary: complete arterial and capillary filling with venous laminar flow
    (d) venous:
        (i) early
        (ii) mid
        (iii) late
4 Side effects (incidence of side effects constant with differing concentrations):
    (a) yellow discoloration of skin
    (b) dark urine
    (c) nausea and vomiting
    (d) red after image
    (e) phlebitis
    (f) syncope
    (g) laryngeal oedema
    (h) anaphylactic shock

Other uses of fluorescein

1 Detection of corneal epithelial defects
2 Applanation tonometry
3 Tear film assessment
4 Hard contact lens fitting
5 Test of lacrimal drainage system patency
6 Seidel's test for aqueous leakage
7 Anterior segment angiography
8 Fluorophotometry

Causes of hyperfluorescence

1 Atrophy of RPE cells (window defect)
2 Dye in subretinal space
3 Dye in RPE detachment
4 Dye leakage from retinal vessels
5 Dye leakage from choroidal or retinal new vessels
6 Dye leakage from optic nerve head in papilloedema
7 Staining of tissues by dye, e.g. drusen

Causes of hypofluorescence

1 Masking by abnormal materials, e.g. blood, melanin, and hard exudates
2 Retinal ischaemia, e.g. retinal capillary closure
3 Choroidal ischaemia
4 Atrophy of vascular tissue, e.g. myopia

Age related macular degeneration (ARMD)

Leading cause of blindness in the Western World. Accounts for 26–30% of all blind registrations in the UK; bilateral asymmetrical disease.
1 Drusen:
   (a) white–yellow lesions at posterior pole
   (b) occur frequently in patients over 60 years
   (c) composed of hyaline material deposited in Bruch's membrane
   (d) may represent reduced efficiency of RPE phagocytosis
   (e) 2 morphological types:
       (i) large, fluffy (soft)
       (ii) small, discrete (hard)
   (f) pathology:
       (i) atrophy of RPE and photoreceptor outer segments
       (ii) thickening and hydrophobicity of Bruch's membrane
       (iii) macrophage invasion of drusen; vascularisation
       (iv) polarity of drusen determines fluorescence
   (g) significance:
       (i) in patients under 50 consider mesangioproliferative glomerulonephritis type II or dominant drusen
       (ii) in senile macular degeneration (SMD), with hyperpigmented large confluent soft drusen, high risk of progression to

subretinal neovascular membranes or SRNVMs (about 9% per year)

2 RPE tears:
  (a) aetiology:
    (i) age related macular degeneration: association with occult SRNVMs
    (ii) photocoagulation
  (b) features:
    (i) acute severe visual loss—a small subset may retain good acuity in spite of subfoveal rip
    (ii) round, asymmetrical elevation of RPE
    (iii) paler area contiguous with and sharply demarcated from darker area
    (iv) ±intraretinal haemorrhage, exudate, serous elevation of retina
    (v) dense hyperfluorescence of paler area; hypofluorescence of darker area
    (vi) high risk of contralateral severe visual loss (37% in first year) as a result of RPE rip or SRNVM

3 Dry ARMD:
  (a) choroidal sclerosis
  (b) large areas of well circumscribed atrophy of RPE, neurosensory retina, and choriocapillaris
  (c) large choroidal vessels prominent

4 Exudative ARMD:
  (a) detachment of retinal pigment epithelium (PED):
    (i) serous, demarcated, yellow to orange, dome shaped elevation of RPE changes if longstanding on angiography, progressively increasing intensity but not area of hyperfluorescence
    (ii) atypical—suggestive of occult SRNVM:
      • notching of PED
      • uneven elevation of PED
      • radial chorioretinal folds surrounding PED
      • intraretinal exudate
      • intraretinal or subretinal blood
      • serous retinal elevation
      • loculated fluid within the retina
      • on angiography irregular filling or hot spot
    (iii) drusen PED:
      • confluent drusen producing pigment epithelial elevation
  (b) subretinal neovascular membrane:
    (i) metamorphopsia ± acute visual loss
    (ii) round/oval green to grey lesion
    (iii) RPE detachment—serous, haemorrhagic, or solid (drusen)
    (iv) loculated fluid within retina if subfoveal
    (v) serous retinal elevation
    (vi) intraretinal and subretinal haemorrhage, occasional intra-vitreal
    (vii) intraretinal exudate
    (viii) later disciform scarring
    (ix) on angiography may be well defined (classic) or not (occult)

Disciform degeneration

Circumscribed scarring at macula as a result of haemorrhage from subretinal neovascular membranes. Subretinal neovascular membranes are stimulated to proliferate as a result of abnormalities of choriocapillaris, Bruch's membrane, RPE, and outer retinal layers.

Causes of subretinal neovascular membranes (SRNVM)

1 Congenital or hereditary:
   (a) rubella retinopathy
   (b) Best's disease
   (c) cone dystrophy
   (d) retinitis pigmentosa
2 Inflammatory:
   (a) presumed ocular histoplasmosis syndrome
   (b) birdshot choroidoretinopathy
   (c) acute multifocal placoid pigment epitheliopathy
   (d) serpiginous choroidopathy
   (e) Harada's disease
   (f) chronic uveitis
   (g) toxoplasmosis
   (h) toxocariasis
3 Vascular:
   (a) Coats' disease
   (b) central or branch retinal vein occlusion
4 Traumatic:
   (a) choroidal rupture
   (b) photocoagulation
   (c) retinal detachment surgery
5 Neoplastic:
   (a) choroidal naevus
   (b) choroidal melanoma
   (c) choroidal haemangioma
   (d) choroidal metastases
   (e) RPE hamartoma
6 Degenerative:
   (a) senile macular degeneration
   (b) myopia (Fuchs' spot)
   (c) angioid streaks
   (d) serpiginous choroidopathy
   (e) optic nerve drusen

Management of ARMD

1 Observe, especially if fellow eye blind
2 Low vision aids
3 Blind/partial sight registration:
   (a) two major prognostic categories of SRNVM (Gass)
   (b) type 1:
       (i) patient age > 50 years
       (ii) membrane between Bruch's membrane and RPE

  (iii) poor prognosis for laser and surgery
  (c) type 2:
      (i) patient age <50 years
      (ii) membrane grows through RPE and ensheathed by proliferating RPE
      (iii) better prognosis for laser and surgery
4 Photocoagulation:
  (a) extrafoveal membrane: macular photocoagulation; study indications for treatment:
      (i) classic SRNVM >200 μm from fovea
      (ii) only 15% of SRNVM fall into this category
  (b) subfoveal membranes: macular photocoagulation; study indications for treatment:
      (i) on angiography, classic SRNVM, well defined borders, <3·5 disc areas in size
      (ii) visual benefit only apparent some years after treatment
5 Treatment still under experimental modalities: surgery to remove SRNVM, radiotherapy, interferon

Angioid streaks

Dehiscences in collagenous and elastic layers of Bruch's membrane, with secondary changes in choriocapillaris and RPE.
1 Features:
  (a) dark irregular lines radiating from optic disc
  (b) may interlink around the optic disc
  (c) irregular paths ending abruptly posterior to the equator
  (d) may cause subretinal neovascularisation
  (e) usually bilateral
  (f) 50% related to systemic disorders of skin, bone, and blood
2 Associations:
  (a) pseudoxanthoma elasticum
  (b) Ehlers–Danlos syndrome
  (c) Marfan's syndrome
  (d) Paget's disease
  (e) sickle cell anaemia
  (f) thalassaemia
  (g) lead poisoning
  (h) acromegaly

Central serous choroidoretinopathy

1 Features:
  (a) unilateral
  (b) M>F, 20–45 years
  (c) often "obsessive" personality
  (d) myopic
2 Symptoms:
  (a) blurring of central vision
  (b) metamorphopsia
  (c) micropsia

3 Signs:
  (a) visual acuity 6/6 to 6/36; often improves with a + 1·00 D lens
  (b) positive paracentral or central scotoma
  (c) red desaturation
  (d) small serous sensory retinal detachment of macula
  (e) sometimes in association with optic disc pit
4 Pathogenesis:
  (a) breakdown of outer blood–retina barrier
  (b) fluid in subretinal space
  (c) sometimes associated with a smaller RPE detachment
5 Fluorescein angiogram: smokestack or inkblot appearance in late venous phase
6 Prognosis:
  (a) 90% spontaneously resolve
  (b) 40% recur
7 Treatment:
  (a) conservative
  (b) photocoagulation if:
      (i) recurrences have left a visual defect
      (ii) duration is longer than 6 months
      (iii) visual impairment in affected fellow eye
           (visual outcome is long term, not modified by photocoagulation)

Cystoid macular oedema

1 Features:
  (a) lack of supporting mechanisms for Henle's layer allows accumulation of extracellular fluid leaking from macular capillaries
  (b) forms flower petal arrangement as a result of radiation of cone fibres
  (c) may develop intraretinal cysts
2 Causes:
  (a) vitreous:
      (i) preretinal membrane formation
      (ii) vitritis
  (b) retina:
      (i) diabetes
      (ii) central or branch retinal vein occlusion
      (iii) macroaneurysms
      (iv) telangiectasia
      (v) hypertension
      (vi) tumours
      (vii) retinitis pigmentosa
      (viii) adrenaline toxicity in aphakia
      (ix) retinitis
      (x) vasculitis
      (xi) Irvine–Gass syndrome
  (c) choroid:
      (i) tumours, especially haemangioma

    (ii) subretinal neovascularisation
    (iii) longstanding uveitis

Irvine–Gass syndrome

1 Cystoid macular oedema occurring after cataract surgery
2 Occurs especially after intracapsular extraction with vitreous loss
3 Of cases, 10–15% are clinically evident
4 Detectable in 90% of cases with angiography
5 Most resolve by 6 months
6 Non-steroidal anti-inflammatory drugs may help

Macular hole

1 Features:
    (a) full thickness retinal hole
    (b) cuff of surrounding subretinal fluid
    (c) deposits at base
2 Causes:
    (a) idiopathic; classification:
        (i) stage 1—impending macular hole loss of foveal depression with yellow spot or halo
        (ii) stage 2—small early hole <500 μm; vitreous attached
        (iii) stage 3—developed hole, about 500 μm with vitreofoveal separation
        (iv) stage 4—complete posterior vitreous detachment
    (b) myopia
    (c) trauma
3 Differential diagnosis:
    (a) large cyst in cystoid macular oedema
    (b) pseudomacular hole: gap in epiretinal membrane
    (c) lamellar hole: partial thickness hole
4 Management: vitrectomy and gas tamponade may be beneficial for stage 2 idiopathic macular holes of less than 6 months' duration; use of agents that promote adhesion, e.g. serum, transforming growth factor β still controversial

Vitreoretinal interface maculopathy

Proliferation of epiretinal membranes; contraction produces macular traction.
1 Types:
    (a) early (cellophaning):
        (i) often no visual symptoms
        (ii) translucent sheen
        (iii) retinal striae
        (iv) slight retinal traction
    (b) late (macular pucker):
        (i) increasing distortion
        (ii) opaque membrane visible
        (iii) macular oedema

2 Causes:
  (a) idiopathic
  (b) retinal detachment surgery (7% of cases)
  (c) photocoagulation (especially excessive panretinal photocoagulation)
  (d) cryotherapy (not as common as photocoagulation)
  (e) central or branch retinal vein occlusion
  (f) diabetic retinopathy
  (g) trauma
  (h) longstanding chorioretinitis
3 Treatment:
  (a) conservative
  (b) surgical:
      (i) membrane peeling
      (ii) useful if vision better than 6/18 and history short
      (iii) full visual recovery uncommon

Choroidal folds

1 Features:
  (a) horizontal parallel folds at posterior pole
  (b) alternating dark and light lines
  (c) fluorescein angiography shows hyperfluorescent crests and hypofluorescent troughs
2 Causes:
  (a) idiopathic (associated with hypermetropia)
  (b) orbital disease:
      (i) dysthyroid eye disease
      (ii) orbital cellulitis
      (iii) orbital tumours
  (c) ocular disease:
      (i) scleral buckling procedures
      (ii) scleritis
      (iii) choroidal tumours
      (iv) ocular hypotony
      (v) ocular trauma
      (vi) papilloedema

Drug induced macular disease

1 Chloroquine:
  (a) uses:
      (i) malaria prophylaxis
      (ii) rheumatoid arthritis
      (iii) systemic lupus erythematosus
  (b) toxicity:
      (i) very few cases with a total dose of < 300 g (250 mg daily for about 3 years)
      (ii) ocular toxicity very unlikely with doses of less than 4 mg/kg per day
      (iii) drug binds to melanin and interacts with nucleic acids

161

    (c) ocular features:
- (i) reversible cornea verticillata
- (ii) premaculopathy
  - reversible
  - scotoma to red targets between 4° and 9° from fixation
- (iii) maculopathy:
  - irreversible
  - may worsen despite withdrawal of drug
  - visual impairment
  - central scotoma
  - central hyperpigmentation with hypopigmented surround (bull's eye)
  - electro-oculogram (EOG) reduced

2 Hydroxychloroquine:
- (a) lower incidence of retinal toxicity than chloroquine
- (b) toxicity:
  - (i) unlikely if cumulative dose does not exceed 200 g (a maximum dose of 600 mg daily is equivalent to 219 g in 1 year)
  - (ii) very unlikely with doses of less than 6·5 mg/kg per day

3 Chlorpromazine:
- (a) major tranquilliser
- (b) rarely causes RPE damage
- (c) toxicity at doses of 2·4 g daily over several years

4 Thioridazine:
- (a) major tranquilliser
- (b) ocular features:
  - (i) retinal pigment clumping and plaques
  - (ii) secondary RPE and choriocapillaris atrophy
- (c) toxicity unlikely at doses of 800 mg/day

5 Tamoxifen:
- (a) antioestrogen used in the treatment of carcinoma of the breast
- (b) ocular features:
  - (i) cystoid macular oedema
  - (ii) RPE atrophy
  - (iii) intraretinal opacities (crystalline deposits)

Causes of a bull's eye maculopathy

1 Chloroquine retinopathy
2 Hydroxychloroquine retinopathy
3 Cone dystrophy
4 Batten's disease
5 Benign concentric annular macular dystrophy

12
HEREDITARY DISORDERS OF THE RETINA AND CHOROID

Hereditary disorders of the retina and choroid account for 33% of blind people in developed countries and 70–90% of blind children.

INVESTIGATIONS OF HEREDITARY RETINAL AND CHOROIDAL DISEASES

1 Visual acuity assessment
2 Colour vision testing:
   (a) pseudoisochromatic plates
   (b) Farnsworth–Munsell 100 hue test
   (c) City University colour plates
   (d) Nagel anomaloscope
   (e) D15 test
3 Adaptometry: measurement of threshold stimulus change with time following retinal bleaching using a Goldmann adaptometer
4 Fluorescein angiography
5 Electrodiagnostic tests
6 Biochemical studies in metabolic disease
7 Genetic studies:
   (a) chromosome morphology
   (b) genetic markers
   (c) disease locus linkage studies using restriction fragment length polymorphism (RFLP)
   (d) biochemical products of abnormal genes
8 Screening:
   (a) family tree
   (b) detection of carriers
9 Prenatal diagnosis:
   (a) amniocentesis
   (b) fetoscopy
   (c) ultrasonography
   (d) chorionic villous sampling

Electro-oculogram (EOG)

1 Indirect measurement of standing potential of eye (6 mV)
2 Uses standardised ocular movements (30° excursion every 12 seconds for 12 minutes)
3 Potential originates in retinal pigment epithelium (RPE)
4 Potential changes with adaptive state
5 Arden index $= \dfrac{\text{Highest potential in photopic state (light peak)}}{\text{Lowest potential in scotopic state (dark trough)}}$

Normal $> 1 \cdot 85$

Electroretinogram (ERG)

1 Recording of potentials in retina under the influence of light
2 Features:
  (a) early receptor potential (ERP): positive deflection originating from outer segment of photoreceptors; response to intense stimulus; potential proportional to stimulus intensity
  (b) a wave: negative deflection originating from inner segment of photoreceptors increasing with stimulus to maximum
  (c) b wave: positive deflection; origin Müller's cells; biphasic in mesopic conditions; b_1 = cone response, b_2 = rod response
  (d) oscillatory potentials: small deflections on b wave; origin bipolar cells
  (e) c wave: positive deflection originating in RPE
3 Types (for differentiation of retinal components):
  (a) flicker: rod ERG—low frequency, low luminance stimuli, dark adapted eye; cone ERG—frequency $> 15/\text{min}$
  (b) dynamic: suppressing rod function with pre-test bleaching
  (c) static: rods—scotopic conditions; cones—photopic conditions
  (d) pattern: response to changing pattern stimuli; small amplitude (2 mV); originating in ganglion cells; useful for macular function

Visually evoked potentials (VEPs)

1 Averaged recording of visual cortex activity in response to light stimulus
2 Latency: 90–114 ms
3 Amplitude: about 10 mV
4 Types:
  (a) flash VEP: response representing function of central 20° of retina
  (b) pattern VEP: response representing function of fovea; response increases with pattern size reduction (60′ to 15′ subtended); indication of visual acuity

Specific management aims in hereditary retinal/choroidal disease

1 Provision of prognosis
2 Specific treatments
3 Genetic counselling
4 Prenatal diagnosis and selective abortion
5 Referral to patient self help groups

Hereditary malformations

1 Macular coloboma: occasionally autosomal dominant
2 Myelinated nerve fibres: asymptomatic; occasionally familial (autosomal dominant or AD; autosomal recessive or AR)
3 Posterior persistent hyperplastic primary vitreous (AR); features:
   (a) retinal folds (especially inferiorly)
   (b) persistent hyaloid artery
   (c) cataract
   (d) vitreous bands
4 Norrie's disease (X linked recessive or XLR); features:
   (a) impaired hearing
   (b) mental handicap
   (c) bilateral congenital blindness
   (d) bilateral retrolental vascular masses
   (e) cataract
   (f) phthisis
5 Incontinentia pigmenti (XL); features:
   (a) lethal to males
   (b) recurrent vesicobullous eruptions
   (c) cutaneous pigmentation
   (d) retrolental mass (dysplastic retina)
   (e) cataract
   (f) optic atrophy
   (g) nystagmus
   (h) strabismus

Vitreoretinal abnormalities

1 Juvenile schisis (XLR); types:
   (a) foveal:
      (i) late onset visual failure (> 20 years)
      (ii) coalescing petaloid pattern of cystoid spaces in nerve fibre layer
      (iii) late macular atrophy
      (iv) associated with peripheral schisis (50%)
   (b) peripheral:
      (i) may be present at birth
      (ii) 50% bilateral and inferotemporal
      (iii) splitting of nerve fibre layer
      (iv) vitreous veils, silver wiring, vitreous haemorrhage
      (v) retinal detachment rare (10%)
2 Wagner's disease (AD); features:
   (a) vitreous degeneration (veils) ("empty vitreous")
   (b) peripheral retinal degeneration (lattice)
   (c) retinal vascular sclerosis
   (d) myopia
   (e) cataract (posterior subcapsular)
   (f) multiple retinal holes plus retinal detachment
3 Stickler's syndrome (AD); features:

    (a) hereditary progressive arthro-ophthalmopathy
    (b) marfanoid habitus
    (c) vitreoretinal degeneration (similar to Wagner's)
4 Goldmann–Favre disease (AR); features:
    (a) night blindness
    (b) foveal schisis
    (c) pigmentary retinal degeneration
    (d) cataract
    (e) extinguished ERG

Disorders of photoreceptors

1 Congenital colour defects:
    (a) red and green defects:
        (i) 8% of white European men
        (ii) 0·4% of white European women   } (XLR)
    (b) blue defects:
        (i) tritanomaly (XLR)
        (ii) tritanopia (AD)
    (c) types:
        (i) anomalous trichomatic individuals:
          • require abnormal mixtures of primary colours
          • normal colour matches appear wrong
          • defects—protanomalous (abnormal red); deuteranomalous (abnormal green); tritanomalous (abnormal blue)
        (ii) dichromatic individuals:
          • require only two primary colours to match other colours
          • accept normal colour matches
          • defects—protanopia (absent red); deuteranopia (absent green); tritanopia (absent blue)
2 Congenital achromatopsia (monochromatism):
    (a) complete rod monochromatism (AR); features:
        (i) complete absence of cones
        (ii) photophobia, nystagmus
        (iii) day blindness, defective colour vision
        (iv) vision reduced (about 6/60 level)
        (v) abnormal photopic ERG
        (vi) variants:
          • incomplete (XLR)
          • blue cone (XLR)
    (b) cone monochromatism (inheritance unknown); features:
        (i) normal rods and only one cone type
        (ii) colour blind
        (iii) good vision
3 Night blindness (nyctalopia):
    (a) congenital stationary night blindness (AD, AR, XLR); features:
        (i) non-progressive night blindness
        (ii) no macroscopic fundal pathology
        (iii) monophasic adaptation
        (iv) reduced scotopic b wave on ERG

    (v) possible defective neural transmission
    (vi) AR, XLR forms associated with myopia
    (vii) XLR form has poor vision
  (b) Oguchi's disease (AR); features:
    (i) occurs in Japanese
    (ii) nyctalopia with slow adaptation
    (iii) grey–white fundus appearing normal after period in dark (Mitzuo phenomenon)

Retinitis pigmentosa

1 Group of progressive disorders of retinal photoreceptor/RPE complex
2 Triad of:
  (a) night blindness
  (b) visual field defect
  (c) typical fundal appearance
3 Symptoms:
  (a) night blindness
  (b) visual difficulty resulting from field loss
  (c) photophobia, glare
  (d) family history
  (e) associated defects
4 Signs:
  (a) early:
    (i) reduced dark adaptation
    (ii) annular scotoma
    (iii) equatorial patchy RPE atrophy and hypertrophy
    (iv) narrowing of retinal vessels
  (b) late:
    (i) tubular fields (2–3°)
    (ii) bone corpuscle pigmentation
    (iii) choroidal atrophy
    (iv) retinal venous sheathing
    (v) drusen
    (vi) waxy disc pallor
5 Associated findings:
  (a) myopia
  (b) keratoconus
  (c) optic disc drusen
  (d) posterior subcapsular lens opacities
  (e) glaucoma
  (f) cystoid macular oedema
6 Investigations:
  (a) EOG: light rise; lost early
  (b) ERG: scotopic mainly affected (amplitude recurrence)
7 Inheritance: varies depending on survey and country:
  (a) AR = 51%
  (b) AD = 26%
  (c) XLR = 23%
8 Prognosis: 25% maintain adequate reading vision

9 Atypical variations:
   (a) sine pigmento: inconspicuous pigmentary changes
   (b) macular type (AD, AR): preceding macular changes
   (c) pericentric/central (AR): possible rod–cone dystrophy
   (d) sectoral (AD):
        (i)   symmetrical, bilateral
        (ii) commonly inferonasal
        (iii) ERG reduced
   (e) unilateral: doubtful existence
   (f) progressive albipunctate dystrophy (AR, AD):
        (i)   night blindness
        (ii) field loss progressive
        (iii) white dots in fundus
        (iv) ERG reduced
   (g) fundus albipunctatus:
        (i)   congenital non-progressive nyctalopia
        (ii) widespread peripheral white dots
   (h) Leber's congenital amaurosis (AD):
        (i)   congenital severe blindness (<6/60)
        (ii) ERG reduced
        (iii) associated with renal abnormalities and deafness
        (iv) variable fundal findings:
              • initially little change
              • salt and pepper fundus
              • late retinitis pigmentosa like picture
              • optic atrophy
        (v)   associated ocular features:
              • nystagmus
              • oculodigital syndrome
              • photophobia
              • cataract
              • keratoconus
              • strabismus

Disorders associated with retinitis pigmentosa (RP)

1 Metabolic disorders:
   (a) Bassen–Kornzweig syndrome (AR): *abetalipoproteinaemia*
        (i)   absence of β-lipoprotein
        (ii) features:
              • early—steatorrhoea, acanthocytosis
              • late—ataxia, RP like fundus
        (iii) treatment:
              • large doses of vitamin A and E
              • decrease intake of long chain fatty acids
              • improvement occurs
   (b) Refsum's disease (AR):
        (i)   phytanic acid storage disease (↓ *phytanic acid oxidase*)
        (ii) features:
              • hypertrophic peripheral neuropathy

- ataxia *cerebral*
- deafness
- cardiomyopathy *+ arrythmia*
- ichthyosis

    (iii) treatment—eliminate phytates (dairy products)
- (c) Batten's disease
- (d) gangliosidoses
- (e) mucopolysaccharidoses

2 Mitochondrial muscle dystrophy:
- (a) results in a chronic, progressive, external ophthalmoplegia
- (b) Kearns–Sayre syndrome:
  - (i) progressive external ophthalmoplegia
  - (ii) pigmentary retinopathy
  - (iii) heart block caused by cardiomyopathy

3 Myotonic dystrophy

4 Neurological disorders:
- (a) ataxia:
  - (i) Friedreich's (AR)
  - (ii) Marie's (AD)
- (b) deafness:
  - (i) Usher's syndrome (AR):
    - 5% of childhood deafness
    - cataracts may occur
  - (ii) Hallgren's syndrome—deafness, ataxia, psychiatric disturbances, and presenile cataract
  - (iii) Alström's syndrome—deafness, obesity, diabetes mellitus, renal impairment, baldness, acanthosis nigricans, raised uric acid and triglycerides, skeletal abnormalities, and hypogonadism
  - (iv) Laurence–Moon–Bardet–Biedl syndrome (AR)—deafness, polydactyly, mental handicap, obesity, and hypogonadism
  - (v) Cockayne's syndrome (AR)—deafness, cataract, dwarfism, mental handicap, and progeria

Causes of pseudoretinitis pigmentosa

1 Infections:
- (a) syphilis retinopathy
- (b) rubella retinopathy

2 Calcium oxalate retinopathy

3 Ocular injury

4 Spontaneous retinal reattachment

5 Drug induced:
- (a) quinine
- (b) phenothiazines

6 Vascular occlusion

Management of retinitis pigmentosa

1 Genetic counselling

2 Referral to self help groups

3 Management of associated ocular findings, e.g. glaucoma and cataract

4 Exclude treatable metabolic disorders
5 (Avoid excessive illumination, which may have a role in disease progression)

Cone dystrophy (AD)

1 Type I:
   (a) reduced photopic vision
   (b) photophobia
   (c) onset 10–30 years
   (d) bull's eye macular appearance
   (e) photopic ERG abnormal
2 Type II:
   (a) more severe disease
   (b) extensive changes (bone spicule)

Sjögren's dystrophy (AR)

1 Features:
   (a) childhood onset
   (b) vision normal initially
   (c) initial dark pigment spot in central macula
   (d) progressive pericentral pigmentation

Butterfly dystrophy (uncertain inheritance)

Butterfly shaped central pigmentation.

Sorsby's dystrophy (AD)

1 Features:
   (a) bilateral
   (b) patients usually 30–50 years of age
   (c) retinal oedema, exudates, and haemorrhage in macular area
   (d) progresses to choroidoretinal atrophy

Familial drusen (AD)

1 Most common flecked macular syndrome
2 Features:
   (a) onset after 20 years
   (b) bilateral, central, yellow lesions
   (c) electrodiagnostic tests normal

Stargardt's disease (AR)

1 Features:
   (a) central visual loss
   (b) onset 10–20 years
2 Types:
   (a) central: atrophic ovoid foveal (beaten bronze) lesion
   (b) central and pericentral:

    (i) pigmentary retinopathy
    (ii) fishtail lesions (white) at posterior pole
(c) central and peripheral:
    (i) pigmentary retinopathy
    (ii) vessel narrowing
    (iii) disc pallor
    (iv) EOG slightly reduced
    (v) ERG—progressive cone loss

Fundus flavimaculatus (AR)

Variant of Stargardt's.
1 Features:
    (a) progressive, powdery, central fishtail lesions at RPE level
    (b) 50% have Stargardt's type fovea

Best's vitelliform dystrophy (AD)

1 Features:
    (a) bilateral
    (b) variable appearance
    (c) average onset 6 years
    (d) abnormal EOG in carriers
2 Stages:
    (a) previtelliform: abnormal EOG
    (b) vitelliform: macular cyst composed of lipofuscin
    (c) pseudohypopyon: cyst absorption reducing colour vision
    (d) vitelliruptive: scrambled egg appearance, reduced vision
    (e) end stage: loss of vision resulting from:
        (i) macular scarring
        (ii) disciform degeneration
        (iii) macular atrophy

Adult vitelliform macular dystrophy (AD)

1 Round/oval, subretinal, yellow, foveal lesions
2 One third to one half disc diameter
3 Bilateral and symmetrical
4 Fourth to fifth decade
5 Minimal symptoms: mild metamorphopsia
6 Lesion fades with time, neovascular membranes rare
7 EOG: normal light peaks

CHOROIDAL DEGENERATIONS

1 Central areolar sclerosis (AR, AD):
    (a) features:
        (i) onset 20–40 years
        (ii) bilateral central atrophy
        (iii) progressive visual loss
        (iv) ERG and EOG are normal

2 Generalised choroidal atrophy (AD): widespread choriocapillaris atrophy
3 Gyrate atrophy (AR):
  (a) deficiency of orthinine ketoacid aminotransferase
  (b) features:
      (i) onset 10–30 years
      (ii) night blindness, tunnel vision
      (iii) patchy, coalescing, progressive, equatorial, choroidal atrophy
      (iv) myopia
      (v) cataract
      (vi) reduced ERG and EOG
      (vii) raised serum ornithine levels
  (c) treatment:
      (i) high dose vitamin B$_6$
      (ii) proline supplementation
4 Choroideraemia (XLR):
  (a) features:
      (i) onset 5–10 years
      (ii) night blindness progressing to blindness
  (b) fundal findings:
      (i) early—granular pigmentary changes
      (ii) late—total choroidal atrophy
  (c) carrier state: midperipheral pigmentary changes which do not progress
5 Degenerative myopia:
  (a) seventh most common cause of blind registration in the UK
  (b) blindness often results in young adulthood
  (c) features:
      (i) cornea—increased corneal diameter
      (ii) trabecular meshwork:
          • chronic open angle glaucoma
          • steroid responsiveness
      (iii) lens—posterior subcapsular opacities
      (iv) vitreous:
          • syneresis and synchysis
          • posterior detachment
          • opacities
      (v) retina:
          • straightening of retinal vessels
          • macular hole
          • peripheral retinal holes and degenerations, e.g. lattice
      (vi) choroid/RPE:
          • pallor
          • tessellation
          • hyperpigmentation at macula
          • lacquer cracks (yellow–white lines representing cracks in Bruch's membrane; 4% of high myopic individuals)
          • subretinal neovascularisation at the macula
          • Foster–Fuchs spot—elevated and varying in colour
      (vii) choroid/sclera—posterior staphyloma

(viii) optic disc:
- pallor
- enlargement—usually caused by optical magnification
- crescent—may encircle the disc, but more commonly temporal; white (scleral); pigmented (choroidal)
- central retinal artery and vein bifurcating on (usually temporal) disc surface (T sign)

STORAGE DISORDERS ASSOCIATED WITH FUNDAL PATHOLOGY

1 Sphingolipidoses:
  (a) Tay–Sachs disease (AR); features:
    (i) normal at birth
    (ii) fatal by 3 years
    (iii) hypotonia, hyperacusis, convulsions
    (iv) cherry-red macular spot (early)
    (v) reduced visually evoked response
    (vi) serum hexosaminidase A level diagnostic
    (vii) ganglion cells laden with membranous cytoplasmic bodies
  (b) Sandhoff's disease (AR); features:
    (i) similar to Tay–Sachs
    (ii) extensive visceral involvement
  (c) sulphated cerebrosidosis (AR):
    (i) group of diseases
    (ii) features:
      - infantile onset
      - ataxia
      - mental handicap
      - grey perifoveal infiltrate
      - fatal disorder
  (d) Niemann–Pick disease (AR):
    (i) group of disorders; most important form is group A (infantile)
    (ii) features:
      - hepatosplenomegaly
      - retarded physical and mental development
      - cherry-red macular spot
      - late optic atrophy
      - foam cells in bone marrow biopsy
2 Batten's disease (AR):
  (a) accumulation of autofluorescent lipopigments in neural, visceral, and somatic tissues
  (b) most important form is juvenile (onset 4–6 years)
  (c) features:
    (i) psychomotor deterioration
    (ii) visual failure
    (iii) increasing white macular spot
    (iv) vessel narrowing
    (v) optic atrophy

(vi) pigmentary disturbance
(vii) vacuolated lymphocytes and abnormal peroxidase activity in blood
(viii) ceroid bodies in skeletal muscle, white blood cells, Schwann cells, and rectal, skin, and conjunctival tissue
3 Cherry-red spot: myoclonus syndrome (AR):
  (a) features:
    (i) myoclonic seizures
    (ii) normal intelligence
    (iii) cherry-red spot (early)
    (iv) deteriorating vision
    (v) ERG normal
    (vi) visual evoked potential reduced
4 Mucopolysaccharidoses (AR):
  (a) extensive accumulation of mucopolysaccharides (MPSs)
  (b) 6 types; distinguished by urinalysis
  (c) features:
    (i) corneal clouding
    (ii) optic atrophy
    (iii) mental handicap
    (iv) physical deformity
  (d) types associated with pigmentary retinopathy:
    (i) MPS 1H—Hurler's syndrome
    (ii) MPS 1S—Scheie's syndrome
    (iii) MPS 2—Hunter's syndrome
    (iv) MPS 3—Sanfilippo's

ALBINISM

1 Failure of melanocyte or melanosome system in varying amounts, producing varying deficiency of melanin
2 Biochemistry:
Phenylalanine → Tyrosine → Dihydroxyphenylalanine (dopa)
$$\downarrow$$
Melanin
3 Enzyme defects:
  (a) tyrosinase negative albinism
  (b) tyrosinase positive albinism

Types of albinism

1 Generalised type: oculocutaneous (AR):
  (a) tyrosinase positive group:
    (i) differentiated by hair bulb incubation in tyrosine solution (producing pigmentation) after age 4 years
    (ii) features:
      • mild, improving with age
      • iris transillumination
      • nystagmus
      • poor vision

- refractive errors
- (b) tyrosinase negative group:
  - (i) features:
    - severe disease
    - photophobic
    - poor vision
    - nystagmus
    - iris transillumination
    - no fundal pigmentation
    - absent foveal reflex
    - refractive errors
    - 90% of fibres decussate at chiasma
    - lateral geniculate body organisation abnormal
    - negative hair bulb test
- (c) yellow mutant group:
  - (i) features:
    - normal skin pigmentation develops
    - ocular changes persist
- (d) Hermansky–Pudlak syndrome:
  - (i) subgroup of tyrosinase negative
  - (ii) associated haemorrhagic diathesis
  - (iii) avoid drugs blocking prostaglandin synthase
- (e) Chediak–Higashi syndrome:
  - (i) features:
    - mild albinism
    - altered immunity, recurrent infections
    - fatal disease
    - neutrophils show large inclusion bodies
    - total lack of RPE pigmentation
  - (ii) treatment—vitamin C may improve leukocyte function

2 Ocular type (XLR):
- (a) confined to eyes
- (b) abnormality of optic cup derived melanocytes
- (c) giant melanosomes in RPE
- (d) carriers:
  - (i) iris transillumination
  - (ii) RPE granularity

3 Partial type (AD):
- (a) albinoid features
- (b) eyes not affected

13
OCULAR TUMOURS

IRIS NAEVUS

1 Slightly elevated discrete pigmented mass
2 Benign, usually spindle A or B cell type
3 Serial observation required
4 Increased incidence in neurofibromatosis type I (Lisch nodules)
5 Cogan–Reese syndrome–diffuse iris naevus

CHOROIDAL NAEVUS

1 Five per cent of adult white Europeans
2 Flat or slightly elevated—less than 2 mm elevation on ultrasonography
3 Oval with indistinct margins with or without overlying drusen
4 Occasionally associated with disciform macular degeneration
5 Usually <5 mm diameter
6 No subretinal fluid
7 No lipofuscin

MALIGNANT MELANOMA OF IRIS

1 Features:
    (a) average age 40–50 years
    (b) ectropion uveae
    (c) pupillary distortion
    (d) neovascularisation
    (e) local lens opacities
    (f) secondary glaucoma
    (g) uveitis
2 Types:
    (a) nodular ⎫
    (b) diffuse ⎬ pigmented or amelanotic; usually spindle A or B
3 Treatment:
    (a) observation
    (b) local resection
    (c) <5% mortality rate
    (d) low recurrence rate even if incompletely excised

MALIGNANT MELANOMA OF CILIARY BODY

1 Fifteen per cent of choroidal melanomas
2 Features:
  (a) late presentation
  (b) lens subluxation
  (c) uveitis
  (d) secondary glaucoma
  (e) sentinel episcleral vessels
  (f) failure of accommodation
2 Types:
  (a) localised (95%)
  (b) diffuse or annular (poor prognosis) (5%)

MALIGNANT MELANOMA OF CHOROID

1 Features:
  (a) average age 50–60 years
  (b) rare in people who are not white Europeans
  (c) may arise in pre-existing naevus
  (d) may contain orange pigmentation (lipofuscin)
  (e) presentation:
     (i) visual field loss
     (ii) macular involvement
     (iii) serous retinal detachment
     (iv) uveitis – masquerading
     (v) secondary glaucoma
     (vi) chance finding
  (f) acoustic hollowness and choroidal excavation on B scan ultra-sonography
2 Types:
  (a) localised
  (b) diffuse (rare, poor prognosis)
  (c) pigmented or amelanotic
3 Spread:
  (a) local
  (b) haematogenous (especially to liver)
4 Histology:
  (a) cellular type:
     (i) spindle A—spindle shaped cells, flattened nucleus, no nucleoli—central chromatin bar
     (ii) spindle B—round/oval nucleus, prominent nucleoli
     (iii) epithelioid—large oval/round cells, eosinophilic cytoplasm, distinct cell border, round nuclei, prominent nucleoli, many mitotic figures
  (b) histological features:
     (i) fascicular—palisading of cells
     (ii) mixed—spindle and epithelioid cells
     (iii) necrotic—cell type not recognisable
5 Features that indicate a poor prognosis:

    (a) large size
    (b) extraocular spread
    (c) presence of epithelioid cells and necrosis
    (d) anteriorly placed tumour
    (e) diffuse tumour
    (f) rupture of Bruch's membrane
    (g) highly pigmented
    (h) raised intraocular pressure

6 Differential diagnosis:
    (a) benign naevus
    (b) metastatic carcinoma
    (c) pigment epithelial hyperplasia
    (d) retinal detachment
    (e) choroidal haemangioma
    (f) disciform degeneration
    (g) congenital ciliary body cyst
    (h) melanocytoma
    (i) astrocytoma
    (j) choroidal haemorrhage/detachment

7 Management: controversial; tailored to patient's requirements:
    (a) observation (until diagnosis made)
    (b) general examination (to exclude metastases)
    (c) enucleation
    (d) photocoagulation
    (e) irradiation, e.g. local plaque, charged particle beam
    (f) local resection
    (g) exenteration (extraocular extension or orbital recurrence)

METASTATIC DEPOSITS

Most common intraocular tumours.

1 Features:
    (a) often multiple
    (b) white, round lesions
    (c) respond to local radiotherapy
    (d) rapid growth (main value of observation)

2 Primary source:
    (a) breast: 75% in women
    (b) lung: 50% in men
    (c) gastrointestinal tract
    (d) kidney
    (e) prostate
    (f) thyroid
    (g) testes

OTHER TUMOURS

1 Choroidal haemangiomas (second most common primary intraocular tumour):

    (a) localised
        (i) red–orange lesion
        (ii) RPE mottling and atrophy
        (iii) serous detachment
    (b) diffuse: associated with Sturge–Weber syndrome
    (c) treatment:
        (i) photocoagulation
        (ii) radiotherapy (very radiosensitive)

2 Haemangioma of iris
3 Juvenile xanthogranuloma:
    (a) yellow–orange accumulations in iris
    (b) may present with spontaneous hyphaema
    (c) in girls
    (d) bilateral in 50%
    (e) 2nd to 4th decade
4 Choroidal osteoma:
    (a) rare
    (b) 20–30% bilateral
    (c) peripapillary
    (d) in white Europeans; more common in women, occurring in third to fourth decade
    (e) pathology: contains bone and haversian systems
5 Combined harmatoma:
    (a) two types: peripapillary and peripheral
    (b) clinical features:
        (i) vascular tortuosity
        (ii) hyperpigmentation
        (iii) slight elevation
        (iv) epiretinal membrane formation
        (v) hard exudate formation
    (c) associated with neurofibromatosis types I and II

TUMOURS OF CILIARY BODY EPITHELIUM

1 Congenital ciliary body cysts
2 Fuchs' adenoma (benign)
3 Medulloepithelioma:
    (a) rare tumour of ciliary epithelium
    (b) benign or malignant
    (c) average age 5 years (range 1–40 years)
    (d) usually locally invasive

RETINAL ASTROCYTOMA

1 Benign
2 Associated with tuberous sclerosis
3 Fifteen per cent bilateral
4 Single or multiple slow growing tumours at or near optic disc or perivascular

5 Usually nodular
6 Translucent, late calcification (mulberry tumour)

RETINAL CAPILLARY HAEMANGIOMAS

1 Features:
   (a) associated with cerebellar haemangioma, renal carcinoma, phaeo-chromocytoma (von Hippel-Lindau syndrome)
   (b) average age 20–30 years
   (c) gradually enlarging orange–red tumour
   (d) feeder artery and draining vein
   (e) leaking vessels produce:
       (i) retinal exudates
       (ii) serous retinal detachment
       (iii) retinal haemorrhage
2 Treatment:
   (a) early detection in at risk patients
   (b) photocoagulation
   (c) cryotherapy

RETINAL CAVERNOUS HAEMANGIOMA

1 Congenital
2 Unilateral
3 Aneurysmal lesions with "cluster of grapes" appearance, in inner retina or optic nerve head
4 Asymptomatic

RETINAL RACEMOSE HAEMANGIOMA

1 Congenital unilateral arteriovenous malformation
2 Enlarged tortuous vessels
3 Affects retina or optic nerve head
4 Associated with midbrain arteriovenous malformation
5 Not hereditary

RETINOBLASTOMA

1 Features:
   (a) tumour of primitive photoreceptor cells
   (b) most common childhood ocular malignancy of eye
   (c) average age at presentation 18 months
   (d) prevalence = 1:20 000; M = F
   (e) increased risk of other tumours especially osteosarcoma
2 Inheritance:
   (a) up to 40% hereditary
   (b) retinoblastoma gene located on the long arm of chromosome 13 close to esterase D gene; levels of esterase used to be used as a genetic marker in some cases

(c) increased incidence with trisomy 13, 21, and deletion of long arm of 13

(d) bilateral cases always inherited

(e) increased risk with increasing paternal age

3 Presentation:
  (a) leukocoria
  (b) strabismus
  (c) secondary glaucoma
  (d) proptosis (especially in developing countries)
  (e) anterior uveitis, hyphaema, pseudohypopyon
  (f) routine examination

4 Appearance:
  (a) endophytic: within vitreous cavity; white/pinkish nodular lesion with surface vessels
  (b) exophytic: growing in subretinal space, usually with retinal detachment

5 Differential diagnosis:
  (a) retinopathy of prematurity
  (b) persistent primary hyperplastic vitreous (anterior or posterior)
  (c) congenital cataract
  (d) toxocariasis/toxoplasmosis
  (e) retinal astrocytoma
  (f) retinal dysplasia
  (g) Coats' disease
  (h) medulloepithelioma
  (i) retinal angiomas
  (j) coloboma
  (k) retinal detachment
  (l) Norrie's disease

6 Histopathology:
  (a) small, closely packed, polygonal cells
  (b) high nuclear/cytoplasmic ratio
  (c) attempted differentiation produces Flexner–Wintersteiner rosettes
  (d) necrosis may produce pseudorosettes
  (e) calcification usually occurs

7 Spread:
  (a) trans-sclerally into orbit
  (b) direct along optic nerve
  (c) via subarachnoid space to CNS
  (d) haematogenous, to bone marrow

8 Features that indicate a poor prognosis:
  (a) metastatic spread
  (b) invasion of orbit or sclera
  (c) extension to resected end of optic nerve
  (d) large tumour
  (e) intraocular complications, e.g. cataract, rubeosis, and pseudo-hypopyon
  (f) poor cellular differentiation with lack of rosettes

9 Diagnosis:
  (a) history and ocular/general examination

    (b) family history and examination of relatives
    (c) imaging: ultrasonography, radiography, and CT scan (look for calcification)
    (d) biochemistry:
        (i) α-fetoprotein and carcinoembryonic antigen
        (ii) aqueous/blood lactate dehydrogenase ratio
        (iii) esterase D levels
    (e) serology: titres of *Toxocara/Toxoplasma* spp.
    (f) gene probes

10 Management:
    (a) of patient:
        (i) ocular examination (bilateral or unilateral)
        (ii) general examination to exclude metastases
        (iii) unilateral: enucleation if large
        (iv) bilateral:
            • radiation
            • cryotherapy
            • photocoagulation
        (v) metastatic: systemic chemotherapy
        (vi) regular follow up in early years
    (b) of family:
        (i) genetic counselling
        (ii) ocular examination of near relatives

14
OCULAR MOTILITY

THE EXTRAOCULAR MUSCLES

1 Features:
  (a) highly specialised striated muscles
  (b) small fibres peripherally:
      (i) slow twitch
      (ii) multiple motor end plates (*en grappe*)
      (iii) graded contractions in absence of action potential
  (c) large fibres centrally:
      (i) fast twitch
      (ii) single motor end plate (*en plaque*)
  (d) small motor unit: 1 axon supplies 6 muscle fibres
  (e) proprioception via nerve V (mesencephalic nucleus)
  (f) specialised muscle spindles
2 The recti:
  (a) all have origin from annulus of Zinn
  (b) 4 cm long
  (c) scleral insertions (spiral of Tillaux):
      (i) medial rectus (MR)—5·5 mm from limbus
      (ii) inferior rectus (IR)—6·5 mm from limbus
      (iii) lateral rectus (LR)—6·9 mm from limbus
      (iv) superior rectus (SR)—7·7 mm from limbus
  (d) tendon length:
      (i) MR—3·0 mm
      (ii) IR—4.7 mm
      (iii) LR—7·2 mm
      (iv) SR—4·3 mm
  (e) muscle length (excluding tendon):
      (i) MR—37·7 mm
      (ii) IR—37·0 mm
      (iii) LR—36·3 mm
      (iv) SR—37·3 mm
  (f) insertion width:
      (i) MR—10·4 mm
      (ii) IR—8·6 mm
      (iii) LR—9·6 mm
      (iv) SR—10·4 mm
  (g) in the primary position of gaze the SR and IR form an angle of 22.5°
      with the ocular axis

(h) nerve supply:
  (i) MR and IR—inferior division of III
  (ii) SR—superior division of III
  (iii) LR: VI
(i) vascular supply:
  (i) LR, SR, LPS (levator palpebrae superioris), and SO (superior oblique) supplied by lateral muscular branch of ophthalmic artery
  (ii) MR, IR, IO (inferior oblique) supplied by medial muscular branch of ophthalmic artery—note that this is the larger branch of the two
  (iii) two anterior ciliary arteries emerge from each tendon of MR, IR, SR; only one emerges from tendon of LR
  (iv) perforating branches of anterior ciliary arteries cross suprachoroidal space to anastomose—lateral and medial long ciliary arteries; this forms the major arterial circle of the iris

3 Superior oblique (SO):
(a) origin from lesser wing of sphenoid superomedial to annulus of Zinn
(b) passes anteriorly above MR
(c) 6 cm long (3 cm muscle, 3 cm tendon)
(d) passes through trochlea 4 cm from origin
(e) 11 mm width insertion behind equator in superotemporal quadrant of globe passing beneath SR
(f) in the primary position of gaze it forms an angle of 54° with the ocular axis
(g) supplied, on its upper surface, by IV

4 Inferior oblique (IO):
(a) origin from orbital floor (vertically below trochlea)
(b) passes obliquely backwards inferior to IR
(c) covered laterally by LR at insertion
(d) 3·7 cm long
(e) in the primary position of gaze it forms an angle of 51° with the ocular axis
(f) 9 mm width insertion behind the equator, 2 mm below and lateral to the macula
(g) supplied by the inferior division of III

Table 14.1 Actions of the different external ocular muscles

Muscle actions	Primary	Secondary
Medial rectus	Adduction	–
Lateral rectus	Abduction	–
Superior rectus	Elevation (maximal in abduction)	Adduction, intorsion (maximal in adduction)
Inferior rectus	Depression (maximal in abduction)	Adduction, extorsion (maximal in adduction)
Superior oblique	Depression (maximal in adduction)	Abduction, intorsion (maximal in abduction)
Inferior oblique	Elevation (maximal in adduction)	Abduction, extorsion (maximal in abduction)

Eye movements

1 Ductions: monocular eye movements:
   (a) adduction
   (b) abduction
   (c) elevation (sursumduction)
   (d) depression (deorsumduction)
   (e) intorsion
   (f) extorsion
2 Versions: binocular eye movements in which the two eyes move synchronously and symmetrically in the same direction:
   (a) dextroversion
   (b) laevoversion
   (c) upgaze
   (d) downgaze
   (e) dextroelevation
   (f) laevoelevation
   (g) dextrodepression
   (h) laevodepression
   (i) dextrocycloversion
   (j) laevocycloversion
3 Vergences: binocular movements in which both eyes move synchronously and symmetrically in opposite directions:
   (a) convergence
       (i) voluntary
       (ii) reflex
           • tonic
           • proximal
           • fusional
           • accommodative
   (b) divergence:
       (i) voluntary
       (ii) reflex (fusional)

AC/A ratio

Accommodative convergence exerted in response to one unit of accommodation (normally 3–5:1).
1 Measured by:
   (a) heterophoria method: prism cover test (PCT) at 6 m and 33 cm
   (b) gradient method: PCT at 6 m then concave lenses inserted in trial frames (up to –3 D) and PCT repeated

Yoke muscles

Muscle pairs acting in each of 6 cardinal positions, e.g. dextroelevation: right SR and left IO:

Right	Left		Right	Left
SR	IO		IO	SR
LR →	MR →	THE YOKE MUSCLES	← MR	← LR
IR	SO		SO	IR

185

Sherrington's law of reciprocal innervation

Increase of innervation and contraction of a muscle is associated with a reciprocal decrease in innervation of the antagonist.

Hering's law of equal innervation

During any conjugate eye movement, equal and simultaneous innervation flows to the yoke muscles.

Hess chart (Lees screen)
Shows the position of the non-fixing eye in all positions of gaze when the other eye is fixing. Based on:
1 Foveal projection
2 Hering's and Sherrington's laws
3 Disassociation of the eyes using complementary colours or a mirror

Schematic representation of Hess chart

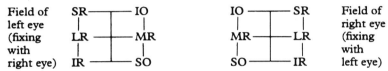

| Field of left eye (fixing with right eye) | SR———IO
LR——MR
IR———SO | IO———SR
MR——LR
SO———IR | Field of right eye (fixing with left eye) |

BINOCULAR FUNCTION

1 Binocular single vision (BSV): the simultaneous use of the two eyes to give a single mental impression in normal conditions of seeing:
  (a) acquired and reinforced in the first 3 years of life
  (b) Worth's classification:
    (i) grade 1 = simultaneous perception:
      • paramacular
      • macular
      • foveal
    (ii) grade 2 = fusion:
      • sensory (the ability to fuse two similar images)
      • motor, i.e. vergence (the ability to align both eyes in order to maintain sensory fusion)
    (iii) grade 3 = stereopsis
  (b) requirements:
    (i) normal retinal correspondence
    (ii) reasonably good vision in each eye
    (iii) the precise coordination of the eyes at all times
    (iv) the ability of the fusional areas of the brain to fuse slightly dissimilar images
  (c) advantages of BSV:
    (i) the field of vision is enlarged
    (ii) elimination of the blind spot
    (iii) binocular visual acuity is slightly greater than monocular

(iv) stereopsis allows very accurate depth perception
2 Horopter: an imaginary surface in space all points of which stimulate corresponding retinal points and are therefore projected to the same locus in space
3 Panum's space: that region around and including the horopter in which BSV can be obtained

Investigation of binocular function

1 Requires the assessment of the presence or absence of:
   (a) retinal correspondence (normal or abnormal)
   (b) suppression
   (c) fusion
   (d) stereopsis
2 Assessment of retinal correspondence:
   (a) Bagolini glasses
   (b) major amblyoscope
   (c) Lang's 2 pencil test
   (d) prism adaptation test
   (e) Worth's 4 lights test
   (f) Bagolini filter bar
   (g) after image test
   (h) binocular visuoscopy
3 Assessment of suppression:
   (a) diplopia tests for peripheral suppression, e.g. Worth's 4 lights test
   (b) major amblyoscope (for peripheral suppression)
   (c) 4 D prism test (for central suppression)
4 Assessment of fusion

Table 14.2 Normal amplitudes

	Near ($\frac{1}{3}$ m) (Δ)	Distance (6 m) (Δ)	Measure with
Convergence	35/40	15	Base out prism
Divergence	15	5	Base in prism
Vertical			
(a) Supravergence	3	3	Base down prism
(b) Infravergence	3	3	Base up prism
Total	6	6	
Cyclovergence (torsional)	(degrees)	(degrees)	
(a) Incyclo	3	3	Major amblyoscope
(b) Excyclo	3	3	
Total	6	6	

5 Assessment of stereopsis:
   (a) qualitative tests:
      (i) Lang's 2 pencil test
      (ii) major amblyoscope
   (b) quantitative tests:
      (i) Titmus test (Wirt)
      (ii) TNO test
      (iii) Lang's stereo test

(iv) Frisby stereo test
(v) Randot test (random dot test)

AMBLYOPIA

Defective visual acuity which persists after correction of any refractive error and removal of any pathological obstacle to vision.
1 Classification:
  (a) stimulus deprivation amblyopia (unilateral or bilateral, complete or partial)
  (b) strabismus
  (c) anisometropic
  (d) ametropic (high bilateral refractive error)
2 Treatment:
  (a) occlusion (total or partial)
  (b) optical penalisation
  (c) cycloplegic drugs

ASSESSMENT OF VISUAL ACUITY

1 Neonates:
  (a) follow a light, face, object (ask mother)
  (b) optokinetic nystagmus
  (c) visually evoked potential
2 At 3–6 months:
  (a) visually directed reaching
  (b) Catford drum
  (c) forced choice preferential looking
3 At 6–18 months:
  (a) Worth's static balls
  (b) Worth's rolling balls
  (c) "hundreds and thousands" pick up test (approximates to 6/24 vision at 33 cm)
4 At 18 months to 3 years:
  (a) Kay's pictures
  (b) Beale–Collins pictures
  (c) Ffookes symbols
  (d) STYCAR 5 letter test (Screening Tests for Young Children And Retards)
5 At 3–5 years (and illiterates):
  (a) Sheridan–Gardiner test
  (b) random dot test
  (c) Sjögren hand test
  (d) Landolt's broken rings
6 Literate children:
  (a) Snellen chart (linear or single optotypes)
  (b) reading types:
    (i) reduced Snellen
    (ii) N (near) test

(iii) J (Jaeger) test

(iv) Maclure's reading books (for children)

(v) Moorfields' bar reading book

(vi) Merrick's reading book

ASSESSMENT OF OCULAR DEVIATION

1 Horizontal and vertical deviations:
- (a) estimation:
  - (i) cover test (cover/uncover, alternate cover)
  - (ii) Hirschberg's method (1 mm deviation = 15 D, e.g. at pupil margin = 30 D)
  - (iii) Krimsky prism reflection test
- (b) measurement:
  - (i) prism cover test (BO or base out for eso, BI or base in for exo, BD or base down for hypertropia)
  - (ii) major amblyoscope
  - (iii) Maddox rod (for distance)
  - (iv) Maddox wing (for close—33 cm)

2 Torsion:
- (a) measurement:
  - (i) 2 Maddox rods
  - (ii) Away's cyclo test
  - (iii) major amblyoscope

NON-PARALYTIC STRABISMUS—ESOTROPIA

Classification

1 Primary esotropia:
- (a) non-accommodative:
  - (i) constant:
    - congenital (infantile) esotropia
    - nystagmus blockage syndrome
    - late onset esotropia
    - myopia associated esotropia
  - (ii) intermittent
    - convergence excess (near esotropia)
    - divergence insufficiency (distance esotropia)
    - cyclic esotropia
- (b) accommodative:
  - (i) constant—partially accommodative esotropia
  - (ii) intermittent
    - fully accommodative esotropia (refractive)
    - accommodative esotropia with convergence excess (non-refractive)

2 Consecutive esotropia:
- (a) features:
  - (i) usually after surgical correction of primary exotropia
  - (ii) rarely spontaneous

(b) management:
  (i) if BSV, surgery early
  (ii) if cosmetic, surgery as required
3 Secondary (symptomatic) esotropia:
  (a) features:
    (i) when there is severe visual loss in one eye or asymmetrical visual loss
    (ii) if congenital or infantile loss, eye may converge or diverge
    (iii) if childhood loss, usually converge
    (iv) if adult loss, usually diverge
  (b) management:
    (i) correct visual loss
    (ii) surgery for cosmesis

Infantile (congenital) esotropia
1 Features:
  (a) onset in first 6 months of life
  (b) large constant angle
  (c) crossed fixation
  (d) alternating or preference
  (e) compensatory head posture (CHP)
  (f) amblyopia infrequent
  (g) emmetropia or low hypermetropia
  (h) dissociated vertical deviation (DVD)
  (i) latent nystagmus
  (j) bilateral inferior oblique overaction (in 20%)
  (k) increased incidence of developmental and neurological abnormalities
2 Management:
  (a) correct any significant ametropia and treat any amblyopia
  (b) early surgery (when stable)

Late onset esotropia
1 Features:
  (a) constant eso with onset at 2–4 years
  (b) large angle
  (c) diplopia may be present (especially early)
  (d) little or no refractive error
  (e) normal retinal correspondence and fusion
2 Management: surgery

Non-accommodative convergence excess esotropia
1 Features:
  (a) intermittent
  (b) controlled for distance, manifest for near
  (c) AC/A ratio normal or low
  (d) emmetropia or low hypermetropia
2 Management:
  (a) correct hypermetropia
  (b) surgery

Non-accommodative divergence insufficiency
1 Features:
   (a) intermittent
   (b) manifest for distance, controlled for near
   (c) no amblyopia
   (d) emmetropia
2 Management:
   (a) try BO prisms if small angle
   (b) surgery
       (note: beware of VI nerve palsy)

Partially accommodative esotropia
1 Features:
   (a) hypermetropia
   (b) onset aged 1–3 years
   (c) deviation greater for near fixation (N > D)
   (d) constant deviation reduced but not eliminated by hypermetropic correction
   (e) more commonly unilateral
   (f) inferior oblique overaction is common
   (g) amblyopia common
2 Management:
   (a) fully correct hypermetropia
   (b) treat amblyopia
   (c) assess BSV
   (d) surgery

Fully accommodative esotropia
1 Features:
   (a) moderate hypermetropia
   (b) BSV usually present
   (c) occasional microtropia
   (d) onset at 2–5 years, often after febrile illness
   (e) intermittent, seen when tired or unwell
   (f) correction of hypermetropia usually eliminates deviation
   (g) deviation about equal for near and distance (N = D)
   (h) AC/A ratio normal
   (i) amblyopia rare
2 Management:
   (a) full correction of hypermetropia
   (b) occlusion if necessary
   (c) orthoptic exercises:
       (i) diplopia recognition
       (ii) control of esotropia without spectacles
       (iii) improvement of BSV without spectacles
   (d) surgery usually unnecessary

Accommodative esotropia with convergence excess
1 Features:
   (a) onset at 2–5 years
   (b) intermittent

(c) high AC/A ratio (6:1 or more)
(d) deviation greater for near (N > D)
(e) often hypermetropic
(f) BSV usually present
(g) occasional microtropia
(h) amblyopia rare
2 Management:
    (a) full correction of hypermetropia or undercorrection of myopia
    (b) occlusion if necessary
    (c) try miotic therapy
    (d) executive bifocals in older children
    (e) orthoptic treatment
    (f) surgery usually necessary

NON-PARALYTIC STRABISMUS—EXOTROPIA

Classification

1 Primary exotropia:
    (a) constant:
        (i) congenital (early onset) exotropia
        (ii) decompensated divergence excess exotropia
    (b) intermittent:
        (i) divergence excess exotropia (distance exotropia)
        (ii) near exotropia
2 Consecutive exotropia (following primary esotropia):
    (a) spontaneous:
        (i) in late childhood or adulthood
        (ii) usually following partially accommodative esotropia with marked hypermetropia
        (iii) weak BSV
        (iv) diplopia if sudden onset of exotropia
    (b) postoperative:
        (i) diplopia if sudden onset
        (ii) usually poor or absent BSV
        (iii) more likely if esotropia was early onset
        (iv) amblyopia
        (v) marked hypermetropia
    (c) management:
        (i) reduce hypermetropic correction
        (ii) base in prisms
        (iii) orthoptic exercises to increase positive fusional amplitude
        (iv) surgery for cosmesis
3 Secondary exotropia:
    (a) features:
        (i) in adults who have developed severe visual loss of one eye
        (ii) occasionally in infants
    (b) management:
        (i) treat cause of visual loss, e.g. cataract extraction
        (ii) preoperative diplopia assessment (prisms, botulinum toxin)
        (iii) cosmetic surgery on defective eye in adults

(iv) defer surgery in children until stable

Congenital exotropia
1 Features:
   (a) onset in first 6 months of life
   (b) uncommon
   (c) angle usually large and constant
   (d) often emmetropic
   (e) can have homonymous fixation
   (f) associated with mental handicap
   (g) nystagmus and DVD occur
2 Management:
   (a) wait until stable
   (b) surgery usually needed

Intermittent divergence excess exotropia
1 Features:
   (a) "true" if greater for distance than for near (D > N)
   (b) "simulated" if similar for distance and near (D = N) (test for near with 3 D sphere)
   (c) onset at 2–5 years
   (d) precipitated by daydreaming, tiredness, illness, alcohol (in adults), bright lights (often closing one eye)
   (e) may have suppression or ARC
   (f) may decompensate
2 Management:
   (a) fully correct myopia, under correct hypermetropia (tinted spectacles may help)
   (b) orthoptic exercises (anti-suppression and to increase fusional convergence)
   (c) trial of botulinum toxin into LR
   (d) most require surgery

Intermittent near exotropia
1 Features:
   (a) older children and adults
   (b) asthenopia for near
   (c) poor convergence
   (d) normal retinal correspondence and fusion
   (e) may be myopic
2 Management:
   (a) fully correct myopia, under correct hypermetropia
   (b) orthoptic exercises (diplopia recognition, increasing fusional convergence)
   (c) base in prisms for near
   (d) surgery if above measures fail

MICROTROPIA

A small angle heterotropia (usually 10 D or less) in which a form of BSV exists.

1 Features:
   (a) often anisometropic
   (b) unequal visual acuities, with mild amblyopia and crowding phenomenon
   (c) fixation:
      (i) central (with manifest deviation on CT)
      (ii) eccentric or parafoveal (no movement on CT)
   (d) binocular function
   (e) stereo tests show positive response with reduced stereo acuity
   (f) diagnosed with 4 Δ test
2 Management:
   (a) correct refractive error
   (b) treat amblyopia
   (c) treat any associated heterophoria

HETEROPHORIA

A latent deviation which becomes apparent when the eyes are dissociated.
1 Types:
   (a) exophoria: most common type:
      (i) convergence insufficiency type (N>D)
      (ii) divergence excess type (D>N)
      (iii) non-specific type (D=N)
   (b) esophoria:
      (i) convergence excess type (N>D)
      (ii) divergence weakness type (D>N)
      (iii) non-specific type (D=N)
   (c) hyperphoria: latent vertical deviation
   (d) cyclophoria: wheel rotation of eye on dissociation:
      (i) incyclophoria
      (ii) excyclophoria
2 Symptoms (often non-specific):
   (a) headaches
   (b) fatigue
   (c) burning, itching, and redness of eyes
   (d) blurred vision relieved by closing one eye
   (e) intermittent diplopia
3 Management:
   (a) if fusion range greater than heterophoria, control should be achieved without treatment (similarly if fast recovery on CT)
   (b) correct refractive error
   (c) esophoria:
      (i) orthoptic treatment to improve fusional divergence
      (ii) miotics
      (iii) bifocals in convergence excess
      (iv) surgery if orthoptic exercises fail or deviation too large
      (v) prisms (BO) only as last resort
      (vi) botulinum toxin into MR
   (d) exophoria:
      (i) orthoptic treatment to improve fusional convergence

      (ii) surgery if deviation too large
      (iii) prisms (BI) (minimum possible) as last resort
      (iv) botulinum toxin into LR
  (e) hyperphoria:
      (i) prisms in small deviations
      (ii) surgery if too large for prisms
      (iii) if mixed phoria correct vertical element first
      (iv) botulinum toxin
  (f) cyclophoria:
      (i) correct any associated vertical phoria
      (ii) surgery if necessary

CONVERGENCE INSUFFICIENCY

1 Types:
  (a) primary: inability to obtain or maintain adequate binocular convergence
  (b) secondary: to a heterophoria, e.g. convergence insufficiency exophoria
2 Features:
  (a) frontal headaches and eye strain with close work
  (b) blurred vision or intermittent diplopia for near fixation
  (c) slight exophoria for near
  (d) poor convergence
  (e) uniocular accommodation better than binocular
  (f) poor positive fusional amplitude
3 Management:
  (a) correct refractive error
  (b) teach diplopia recognition
  (c) exercises to improve binocular convergence
  (d) exercises to improve relative positive convergence
  (e) teach voluntary convergence

ANOMALIES OF ACCOMMODATION

1 Accommodative spasm:
  (a) features:
      (i) associated with excessive close work
      (ii) ill fitting or incorrect spectacles
      (iii) asthenopia
      (iv) pseudomyopia (up to 20 D)
      (v) constricted pupils
      (vi) esotropia for distance and occasionally for near
  (b) aetiology:
      (i) undercorrected hypermetropia
      (ii) exotropia
      (iii) organic causes, e.g. cholinergic drugs, morphine, alcohol
      (iv) functional, especially young women
  (c) management:

      (i)   cycloplegic refraction and full correction of hypermetropia
      (ii) treatment with atropine for 4 weeks or more
     (iii) stop close work
     (iv) treat any underlying cause

2 Accommodative insufficiency:
   (a) features:
       (i)   asthenopia
      (ii) blurred near vision
     (iii) exophoria
     (iv) may have reduced convergence
   (b) aetiology:
       (i)   presbyopia
      (ii) disturbance of AC/A ratio as a result of correction of high ametropia
     (iii) after infective illnesses
     (iv) ocular trauma
      (v) drugs such as anticholinergics and antidepressants
   (c) management:
       (i)   remove precipitating factors
      (ii) correct significant refractive error
     (iii) may require reading spectacles
     (iv) treat any exophoria and convergence deficiency

3 Accommodative fatigue:
   (a) features:
       (i)   accommodation initially sufficient then deteriorates
      (ii) similar to, but less severe than, accommodative insufficiency
   (b) aetiology:
       (i)   ill health
      (ii) overwork
     (iii) stress
   (c) management:
       (i)   correct significant refractive error
      (ii) treat any convergence insufficiency
     (iii) often resolves spontaneously

4 Accommodative paralysis:
   (a) features:
       (i)   no accommodation possible
      (ii) blurred vision
     (iii) micropsia
     (iv) diplopia
   (b) aetiology:
       (i)   traumatic paralysis of ciliary muscle (usually with traumatic mydriasis)
      (ii) closed head injuries (including whiplash)
     (iii) drugs, e.g. anticholinergics (especially atropine)
     (iv) nerve III palsy
      (v) midbrain disease, e.g. pinealoma
   (c) management:
       (i)   treat underlying cause
      (ii) correct refractive error

(iii) give middle and near vision addition
(iv) BI prisms may be needed

"A" AND "V" PATTERNS

Changes in the horizontal deviation of the eyes as they move from 30° upgaze to 30° downgaze.
1 Types:
  (a) "A" esotropia: increase in eso on upgaze
  (b) "A" exotropia: increase in exo on downgaze
  (c) "V" esotropia: increase in eso on downgaze
  (d) "V" exotropia: increase in exo on upgaze
    (change of 10 D or more for A pattern, 15 D or more for V pattern)
2 Features:
  (a) V patterns are more common in eso deviations
  (b) A patterns are more common in exo deviations
  (c) may have compensatory head posture
3 Possible aetiologies:
  (a) abnormal actions of horizontal recti in up/downgaze
  (b) abnormal actions of the cyclovertical muscles, i.e. IO, SO, IR, SR
4 Surgical management:
  (a) for cosmesis
  (b) to increase field of BSV

PARALYTIC STRABISMUS

A congenital or acquired incomitant deviation of the visual axes resulting from limitation of ocular movement.
1 Types:
  (a) neurogenic
  (b) mechanical
  (c) myogenic

Neurogenic strabismus

1 Unilateral nerve palsies:
  (a) third cranial nerve palsies
  (b) fourth cranial nerve palsies
  (c) sixth cranial nerve palsies
2 Single muscle palsies:
  (a) medial rectus:
    (i) rare
    (ii) differentiate from atypical Duane's
    (iii) exotropia (N > D)
    (iv) face turns to opposite side
  (b) inferior rectus:

     (i) rare
     (ii) differentiate from mechanical restriction
     (iii) hypertropia and slight exotropia
     (iv) head tilt to opposite side, face turn to affected side, chin down
  (c) superior rectus:
     (i) rare
     (ii) underaction common in a V esotropia
     (iii) hypotropia (D>N) and slight exotropia
     (iv) chin up with head tilt and face turn to affected side
  (d) inferior oblique:
     (i) very rare
     (ii) differentiate from Brown's syndrome ("A" pattern—negative forced duction test muscle sequelae)

3 Bilateral nerve palsies:
  (a) bilateral nerve VI palsy:
     (i) large alternating esotropia (D>N) with crossed fixation
     (ii) no BSV possible
     (iii) sequelae—bilateral contracture of MR
  (b) bilateral nerve IV palsy:
     (i) V esotropia if acquired
     (ii) extorsion and hypertropia (N>D)
     (iii) usually asymmetrical with hypertropia in primary position on more affected side
     (iv) hypertropia may reverse between laevodepression and dextrodepression
     (v) chin down if symmetrical
     (vi) head tilt to side of more affected eye if asymmetrical
     (vii) small field of BSV (if any)
     (viii) sequelae—bilateral overaction of IR

Management of neurogenic strabismus
1 Congenital palsies:
  (a) surgery if large CHP or manifest strabismus
  (b) delay surgery until 4–5 years old
  (c) in adults, no treatment if asymptomatic
2 Acquired palsies:
  (a) exclude treatable cause
  (b) wait until stable (6 months)
  (c) prisms if small deviation or medically unfit
  (d) botulinum toxin to antagonist to prevent contracture and aid diagnosis
3 Surgical principles:
  (a) aim to relieve symptoms
  (b) increase field of BSV (mostly in primary position and in downgaze)
  (c) weaken the ipsilateral antagonist
  (d) strengthen the palsied muscle (if some action remains) or provide motive force in the direction of action of palsied muscle (e.g. Knapp procedure)
  (e) weaken the overacting yoke muscle

Mechanical strabismus

1 Features:
  (a) ductions and versions are equally limited (in neurogenic palsies, versions are usually less than ductions)
  (b) movement often limited in opposite directions of gaze
  (c) muscle sequelae are confined to overaction of contralateral eye in the direction of the limitation of movement
  (d) abnormal movement patterns may result
  (e) saccadic velocity is normal until the point of mechanical restriction is reached
  (f) forced duction test shows restricted passive movements
  (g) globe retraction and rise in intraocular pressure can occur on attempted movement against the restriction
2 Types:
  (a) congenital:
      (i) strabismus fixus—fibrosis and contracture of both MRs; marked esotropia
      (ii) generalised fibrosis syndrome—ptosis and marked bilateral downwards deviation
      (iii) congenital adherence syndromes, e.g. abnormal fascial connections
      (iv) Brown's syndrome
  (b) acquired:
      (i) dysthyroid eye disease—myopathic and later mechanical restriction (usually IR, MR, and SR)
      (ii) orbital injuries, e.g. blow out fractures
3 Management:
  (a) no treatment if asymptomatic or cosmetically acceptable
  (b) prisms
  (c) botulinum toxin to contralateral synergist
  (d) surgery:
      (i) to produce or enlarge field of BSV in straight ahead and downgaze positions
      (ii) to improve cosmesis
      (iii) to reduce any anomalous ocular movements
      (iv) to improve compensatory head posture
      (v) recess tight muscles
      (vi) weaken overacting contralateral synergists

Myogenic strabismus

1 Types:
  (a) myasthenia gravis
  (b) dysthyroid myopathy
  (c) ocular myopathies
  (d) ocular myositis
2 Management:
  (a) treat underlying disease
  (b) surgery usually contraindicated for both ophthalmoplegia and ptosis (risk of corneal exposure)

  (c) relieving prisms
  (d) occlusion to overcome diplopia
  (e) ptosis props

SPECIAL OCULAR MOTILITY SYNDROMES

Brown's syndrome (superior oblique tendon sheath syndrome)
1 Features:
  (a) congenital or acquired in early childhood
  (b) limitation of active and passive elevation in adduction
  (c) down drift of affected eye in adduction (palpebral fissure may widen)
  (d) "V" pattern common
  (e) unilateral or bilateral 10% bilat.
  (f) if unilateral, CHP of chin elevation, and head tilt to affected side
  (g) diagnosed with forced duction test
  (h) may "click"
  (i) often spontaneously improves in late childhood or early teens
  (j) occasionally acquired in adulthood
2 Aetiology:
  (a) congenital:
    (i) tight SO anterior tendon sheath
    (ii) short SO muscle and tendon
    (iii) nodule on SO tendon
    (iv) anomalous innervation
  (b) acquired:
    (i) inflammation
    (ii) trauma
    (iii) SO plication
3 Management:
  (a) if congenital, most are compensated or improve spontaneously
  (b) if marked CHP or decompensation, consider surgery
  (c) if acquired, local steroids or prisms may help

Duane's retraction syndrome
1 Brown's classification:
  (a) type A:
    (i) reduced or absent abduction in one eye with face turn to that side
    (ii) widening of palpebral fissure on abduction
    (iii) narrowing of palpebral fissure and retraction of globe on adduction
    (iv) less marked limitation of adduction
    (v) poor convergence
  (b) type B: limited abduction but normal adduction
  (c) type C:
    (i) adduction more limited than abduction
    (ii) face turn to the opposite side
    (iii) exotropia

(unilateral or bilateral, A or V patterns seen)
(can have associated skeletal, facial, and neural abnormalities)
2 Huber's classification:
   type:
     (i) limitation of abduction
     (ii) limitation of adduction
     (iii) limitation of abduction and adduction
3 Ocular associations:
  (a) colobomas
  (b) heterochromia iridis
  (c) lens opacities
  (d) microphthalmos
  (e) persistent pupillary membrane
4 Possible aetiologies:
  (a) congenital:
     (i) aplasia or dysplasia of VI nerve nucleus
     (ii) more generalised brainstem dysplasia
     (iii) mechanical abnormalities of horizontal recti
  (b) acquired:
     (i) excessive lateral rectus resection
     (ii) localised inflammation
     (iii) orbital trauma
5 Management:
  (a) conservative (the majority)
  (b) surgical only if:
     (i) large CHP
     (ii) decompensation
     (iii) large strabismus

Möbius' syndrome

1 Features:
  (a) rare, congenital
  (b) aplasia of VI, VII, and occasionally IX and XII cranial nerve nuclei
  (c) horizontal gaze palsies
  (d) lower facial muscles often spared
  (e) high refractive errors are common
  (f) mental handicap
  (g) deafness
  (h) pectoral muscle hypoplasia
  (i) limb malformations
2 Management:
  (a) correct significant refractive errors
  (b) treat amblyopia
  (c) avoid surgery unless cosmetically unacceptable strabismus

Double elevator palsy

1 Features:
  (a) unilateral, congenital
  (b) caused by ipsilateral paresis of SR and IO

  (c) restriction of elevation in abduction and adduction
  (d) hypotropia with pseudoptosis
  (e) chin up CHP
2 Management:
  (a) conservative
  (b) surgical only if:
      (i) gross CHP
      (ii) large strabismus

Botulinum toxin

Potent neurotoxin; prevents release of acetylcholine from motor nerve terminals; onset of functional effect is 2 or 3 days post injection; functional effect usually lasts 2–4 months, occasionally long term.
1 Uses:
  (a) predictor of postoperative diplopia or BSV
  (b) nerve palsies
  (c) restrictive myopathies; dysthyroid, or post retinal detachment surgery
  (d) nystagmus
  (e) cases where surgery contraindicated or not preferred
  (f) consecutive exotropia or esotropia
  (g) secondary strabismus
  (h) blepharospasm

15
NEURO-OPHTHALMOLOGY

OPTIC NERVE (II)

1 Features:
    (a) 45 mm long:
        (i) 1 mm intraocular
        (ii) 30 mm intraorbital
        (iii) 6 mm in optic canal
        (iv) 10 mm intracranial
    (b) contains 10^6 myelinated fibres
    (c) myelinated only up to lamina cribrosa
    (d) disc composed of 50% glial tissue, 50% ganglion cell axons
2 Relations:
    (a) embraced by muscle cone
    (b) ciliary ganglion lies laterally
    (c) orbital portion crossed over by:
        (i) nasociliary nerve
        (ii) ophthalmic artery
3 Blood supply:
    (a) pial vessels:
        (i) ophthalmic artery
        (ii) internal carotid artery
        (iii) anterior cerebral artery
    (b) branches of central retinal artery
    (c) posterior ciliary arteries

OPTIC CHIASM

1 Features:
    (a) decussation of nasal fibres
    (b) lower nasal fibres loop forward into opposite optic nerve (anterior knee of Willbrand)
2 Relations:
    (a) chiasma lies above sella in 80% (fixed); anteriorly in 10% (prefixed); posteriorly in 10% (postfixed)
    (b) inferior: diaphragma sellae
    (c) superior: lamina terminalis

(d) anterior: anterior cerebral and communicating arteries
(e) posterior: pituitary stalk
(f) lateral: internal carotid artery
3 Blood supply:
  (a) internal carotid artery
  (b) anterior cerebral artery

OPTIC TRACT

1 Features:
  (a) continuation of optic pathway
  (b) projects to:
    (i) lateral geniculate body (visual fibres)
    (ii) both pretectal nuclei (light reflex fibres)
    (iii) superior colliculus (ocular reflex movements)
2 Relations:
  (a) anterolateral: anterior perforated substance
  (b) posteromedial: pituitary stalk
  (c) inferior: posterior cerebral artery
3 Blood supply:
  (a) anterior choroidal artery
  (b) posterior communicating artery

LATERAL GENICULATE BODY

1 Features:
  (a) receives optic tract
  (b) contains synapses
  (c) saddle shaped
  (d) 6 layers centred on hilum
  (e) crossed fibres project to layers 1, 4, 6
  (f) uncrossed to layers 2, 3, 5
  (g) projects to visual cortex
2 Blood supply:
  (a) posterior communicating artery
  (b) anterior choroidal artery

OPTIC RADIATION

1 Features:
  (a) myelinated nerve fibres
  (b) connecting lateral geniculate body and occipital cortex
  (c) passes in posterior limb of internal capsule
  (d) passes forwards and laterally anterior to lateral ventricle
  (e) lower fibres sweep forward into temporal lobe (Meyer's loop)
2 Blood supply:
  (a) anterior choroidal artery
  (b) deep optic branches of middle cerebral artery
  (c) perforating vessels of calcarine artery (branch of posterior cerebral artery)

VISUAL CORTEX

1 Features:
   (a) medial aspect of occipital lobe
   (b) above and below calcarine fissure
   (c) extends laterally to lunate sulcus
   (d) characterised by stria of Gennari
   (e) macula represented posteriorly
   (f) upper gyrus represents lower field
   (g) 6 layers:
      (i) laminar zonalis
      (ii) outer granular
      (iii) laminar pyramidalis
      (iv) inner granular
      (v) ganglion layer
      (vi) laminar multiformis
2 Blood supply:
   (a) calcarine branch of posterior cerebral artery
   (b) some middle cerebral supply to occipital pole

OCULOMOTOR NERVE (III)

1 Features:
   (a) motor to superior, inferior, and medial recti
   (b) motor to inferior oblique and levator palpebrae superioris
   (c) parasympathetic supply to ciliary body and sphincter pupillae
2 Nuclei:
   (a) paired subnuclei to individual muscles
   (b) at level of superior colliculus
   (c) unpaired caudal subnucleus to levator palpebrae superioris
   (d) pupillomotor nucleus (Edinger–Westphal)
   (e) superior rectus subnucleus supplies contralateral muscle
3 Fasciculus:
   (a) passes ventrally through red nucleus
   (b) emerges into interpeduncular fossa
   (c) between superior cerebellar and posterior cerebral arteries
4 Nerve:
   (a) passes forward below optic tract
   (b) lateral to posterior communicating artery
   (c) enters lateral wall of cavernous sinus
   (d) receives sympathetic supply from internal carotid plexus
   (e) divides into upper and lower divisions
   (f) passes through superior orbital-fissure (within tendinous ring)
   (g) upper division supplies:
      (i) superior rectus
      (ii) levator palpebrae superioris
   (h) lower division supplies:
      (i) inferior and medial recti
      (ii) inferior oblique (with parasympathetic branch to ciliary ganglion)

TROCHLEAR NERVE (IV)

1 Features:
   (a) pure motor nerve
   (b) supplies superior oblique
   (c) longest cranial nerve (7·5 cm)
   (d) only cranial nerve to emerge dorsally
2 Nucleus:
   (a) in dorsal midbrain
   (b) at level of inferior colliculus
3 Fasciculus:
   (a) passes dorsally
   (b) decussates
   (c) emerges below inferior colliculus
4 Nerve:
   (a) passes round midbrain
   (b) between posterior cerebral and superior cerebellar arteries
   (c) passes beneath free edge of tentorium
   (d) enters lateral wall of cavernous sinus
   (e) enters orbit via superior orbital fissure (outside tendinous ring)
   (f) passes medially along orbital roof to superior oblique

TRIGEMINAL NERVE (V)

1 Features:
   (a) sensory to face and eye
   (b) motor to muscles of mastication
2 Nuclei:
   (a) mesencephalic (midbrain): proprioception
   (b) sensory (pontine): light touch, pressure
   (c) spinal (medulla to cervical spine): pain, temperature
   (d) motor (pontine)
3 Nerve:
   (a) emerges from ventral pons
   (b) large sensory root
   (c) small motor root
   (d) passes below tentorium to ganglion
4 Ganglion:
   (a) cell bodies of sensory cells (except proprioception)
   (b) extradural in Meckel's cave
   (c) receives:
       (i) ophthalmic division
       (ii) maxillary division
       (iii) mandibular division
5 Ophthalmic division (Va):
   (a) in lateral wall of cavernous sinus
   (b) divides into:
       (i) lacrimal nerve ⎫ enter orbit via superior orbital fissure
       (ii) frontal nerve ⎬ (outside tendinous ring)
       (iii) nasociliary nerve: enters orbit inside tendinous ring

    (c) supplies sensation to upper face including eye
    (d) 5 branches of nasociliary nerve:
        (i) sensory root of ciliary ganglion
        (ii) 2–3 long ciliary nerves
        (iii) posterior ethmoidal nerve
        (iv) anterior ethmoidal nerve
        (v) infratrochlear nerve
6 Maxillary division (Vb):
    (a) lies in cavernous sinus
    (b) exits cranium via foramen rotundum
    (c) sensory supply to middle of face including inferior conjunctiva
7 Mandibular division (Vc):
    (a) leaves cranium via foramen ovale
    (b) sensory to inferior face
    (c) motor to muscles of mastication

ABDUCENT NERVE (VI)

1 Features: motor to lateral rectus
2 Nucleus:
    (a) near midline in lower pons
    (b) beneath facial colliculus
3 Fasciculus:
    (a) passes ventrally
    (b) exits in pontomedullary groove
4 Nerve:
    (a) passes upward through cisterna pontis
    (b) pierces dura
    (c) passes over apex of petrous bone
    (d) enters cavernous sinus
    (e) enters orbit through superior orbital fissure
    (f) lies within the tendinous ring
    (g) passes laterally to supply lateral rectus

FACIAL NERVE (VII)

1 Features:
    (a) motor to:
        (i) muscles of facial expression
        (ii) stylohyoid
        (iii) posterior belly of digastric
        (iv) stapedius
    (b) secretomotor to lacrimal and salivary glands
    (c) taste to anterior $\frac{2}{3}$ of tongue
2 Nucleus:
    (a) in lower pons
    (b) beneath floor of fourth ventricle
3 Fasciculus:
    (a) passes round abducent nucleus

   (b) exits ventrally from pontomedullary junction
4 Nerve:
   (a) enters internal auditory canal
   (b) geniculate ganglion contains cell bodies of chorda tympani (taste)
   (c) branches within cranium:
      (i) chorda tympani
      (ii) greater superficial petrosal nerve
      (iii) nerve to stapedius
      (iv) branches to tympanic plexus
   (d) exits from stylomastoid foramen
   (e) initial branches:
      (i) posterior auricular nerve
      (ii) tympanic nerve
   (f) branches in parotid gland:
      (i) temporal
      (ii) zygomatic
      (iii) buccal
      (iv) mandibular
      (v) cervical

CILIARY GANGLION

1 Features:
   (a) small parasympathetic ganglion (3 mm long)
   (b) lies 1 cm from optic foramen
   (c) between optic nerve and lateral rectus
   (d) contains parasympathetic synapse
2 Receives:
   (a) long sensory root from nasociliary nerve
   (b) short parasympathetic root from Edinger–Westphal nucleus of nerve III (motor to ciliary body and sphincter pupillae)
   (c) slender sympathetic root (supply to vasculature and dilator pupillae)
3 Branches: 6–7 short ciliary nerves to globe

PUPILLOCONSTRICTOR PATHWAY

1 Afferents pass in optic nerve and tract
2 Synapse in the pretectal nucleus
3 Project to both Edinger–Westphal nuclei *bilat.*
4 Efferents pass in nerve III
5 Lie dorsally and laterally in nerve
6 Pass with branch to inferior oblique
7 Synapse in ciliary ganglion
8 Postganglionic fibres pass in short ciliary nerves to sphincter pupillae

PUPILLODILATOR PATHWAY

1 Sympathetic nervous system
2 Originates in posterior hypothalamus

3 Descends to T1 level (ciliospinal centre of Budge)
4 Synapses in lateral horn
5 Efferent exits with the ventral root
6 Leaves the spinal nerve in the white ramus
7 Enters the sympathetic chain
8 Ascends and synapses in the superior cervical ganglion
9 Postganglionic fibres pass in carotid plexus
10 Transfers to Va in cavernous sinus
11 Passes via long ciliary nerves to dilator muscle

HORIZONTAL GAZE CENTRE

1 Situated in paramedian pontine reticular formation (PPRF)
2 At level of nerve IV nucleus
3 Controls horizontal gaze to ipsilateral side
4 Projects to:
   (a) ipsilateral nerve IV nucleus
   (b) contralateral nerve III nucleus (via contralateral medial longitudinal fasciculus)
5 Saccades generated from contralateral premotor frontal cortex
6 Pursuits generated from ipsilateral occipital cortex

VERTICAL GAZE CENTRE

1 Poorly understood
2 Pretectal and rostral mesencephalic reticular formation
3 Acts bilaterally

VERGENCE CENTRE

1 Ill defined area
2 Similar to vertical gaze centre
3 Defects associated clinically with vertical gaze palsies

MEDICAL LONGITUDINAL FASCICULUS (MLF)

1 Near midline
2 Extending from anterior horn cells of spinal cord to thalamus
3 Connects:
   (a) oculomotor nuclei
   (b) gaze centres

OCULAR MOVEMENTS

1 Saccade:
   (a) refixation movement
   (b) latency 200 ms
   (c) velocity 200–300°/s (fast)
   (d) controlled by:

        (i) frontal cortex
        (ii) superior colliculus
  (e) defects:
        (i) delayed
        (ii) slow
        (iii) hypermetric (overshoot)
        (iv) hypometric (undershoot)
  (f) tests:
        (i) refixation
        (ii) rotation
        (iii) calorics
        (iv) optokinetic nystagmus (fast saccadic return phase)

2 Pursuits:
  (a) conjugate movement
  (b) maintaining foveal fixation
  (c) latency 125 ms
  (d) velocity <50°/s (relatively slow)
  (e) controlled by posterior parietal lobe
  (f) defect: reduced (saccadic pursuit)
  (g) tests:
        (i) doll's head
        (ii) rotation
        (iii) optokinetic nystagmus (smooth pursuit phase)

3 Vergence:
  (a) disjunctive movement
  (b) maintaining foveal fixation on object approach
  (c) latency 160 ms
  (d) velocity <20°/s (slow)
  (e) controlled:
        (i) frontal and occipital lobes
        (ii) possibly midbrain centre
  (f) types:
        (i) voluntary
        (ii) accommodative
        (iii) proximal induced
        (iv) tonic
        (v) fusional
  (g) test: look from distance to near according to type

4 Vestibulo-ocular movements:
  (a) smooth conjugate movement
  (b) maintains steady gaze during head movement
  (c) latency of 10–100 ms
  (d) peak velocity 300–400°/s
  (e) utricle and saccule respond to rectilinear acceleration
  (f) semicircular canals respond to rotational acceleration
  (g) mediated by vestibular nuclei projecting to PPRF
  (h) also input from neck proprioceptors
  (i) defects cause oscillopsia
  (j) tests:
        (i) caloric

    (ii) rotation
    (iii) doll's head

EMBRYOLOGY OF THE VISUAL PATHWAY

1 Primitive optic vesicle (neuroectodermal)
2 Forms as diverticulum from diencephalon
3 Proximal part forms stalk
4 Distal part invaginates to form optic vesicle
5 Optic vesicle forms retina
6 Ganglion cell axons converge and invade optic stalk
7 Medullation of axons proceeds in retrograde direction
8 Mesoderm forms dura, arachnoid, and pia

THE PUPILS

Pupil examination

1 Size, symmetry, shape
2 Reactions (brisk, sluggish)
3 Direct reaction
4 Consensual reaction
5 Near reaction (accommodation)
6 Relative afferent pupillary defect
7 Associated ocular examination, ocular movements, upper lid position, ophthalmoscopy

Pupil abnormalities

1 Essential anisocoria:
   (a) up to 20% prevalence in normal population
   (b) unknown cause
   (c) normal pupil reflexes
2 Persistent pupillary fibres:
   (a) congenital
   (b) remnants of pupillary membrane
3 Iris coloboma:
   (a) congenital
   (b) total or partial
   (c) pigment frill present
4 Corectopia:
   (a) congenital displacement of pupil
   (b) associated with peripheral anterior synechiae
5 Polycoria:
   (a) multiple true pupils
   (b) rare
6 Acquired pupil irregularity:
   (a) posterior synechiae
   (b) traumatic mydriasis

    (c) iris melanoma
    (d) sphincter infarction (acute angle closure glaucoma)
    (e) iridectomy
    (f) iris prolapse
    (g) iridodialysis

7 Horner's syndrome:
    (a) features:
        (i) ptosis (2 mm only)
        (ii) miosis
        (iii) preganglionic type associated with anhidrosis of upper face
        (iv) iris heterochromia (if congenital or longstanding)
    (b) causes:
        (i) congenital
        (ii) interruption of sympathetic pathway (via T1)
        (iii) thalamic, internal capsule, or brainstem lesion, e.g. disseminated sclerosis, glioma, vascular lesions
        (iv) cervical cord lesions, e.g. syringomyelia, glioma, ependymoma
        (v) T1 root lesions, e.g. Pancoast's tumour, cervical rib, avulsion injury
        (vi) cervical sympathetic chain lesions, e.g. Hodgkin's disease, carotid aneurysm, carotid body tumour
        (vii) internal carotid artery or cavernous sinus lesions
    (c) tests:
        (i) hydroxyamphetamine 1% drops dilate pupil only in preganglionic lesion
        (ii) adrenaline 0·1% drops dilate pupil in postganglionic lesions

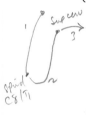

8 Tonic pupil (Adie's):
    (a) young adults (F:M, 2:1)
    (b) dilated pupil (later miosed)
    (c) tonic reaction to light and accommodation but light–near dissociation
    (d) sectorial vermiform movements
    (e) constricts with 0·125% pilocarpine or 2·5% methacholine
    (f) possibly postviral degeneration of ciliary ganglion
    (g) associated with hyporeflexia (Holmes–Adie syndrome)

9 Argyll Robertson pupil:
    (a) bilaterally small irregular pupils
    (b) light–near dissociation
    (c) causes:
        (i) syphilis
        (ii) diabetes mellitus
        (iii) encephalitis

10 Parinaud's syndrome:
    (a) bilateral mid-dilated pupils
    (b) light–near dissociation
    (c) convergence retraction nystagmus
    (d) poor upgaze
    (e) staring facies (Collier's sign)
    (f) causes:

     (i) pinealoma

     (ii) teratoma of pineal gland

     (iii) multiple sclerosis

     (iv) vascular lesions

11 Nerve III palsy (complete):
- (a) dilated fixed pupil
- (b) abducted and slightly depressed eye
- (c) ptosis

12 Afferent pupil defect (Marcus Gunn pupil):
- (a) normal sized pupils
- (b) swinging light test used to elicit sign
- (c) caused by optic nerve or severe retinal disease

13 Drug induced pupil abnormality:
- (a) common cause
- (b) topical:
  - (i) cycloplegics
  - (ii) mydriatics
  - (iii) miotics
- (c) systemic:
  - (i) constricted by opiates
  - (ii) dilated by anticholinergics, antidepressants, amphetamines

14 Disorders of light–near dissociation:
- (a) features:
  - (i) absent or reduced light reaction
  - (ii) near reaction present
- (b) causes:
  - (i) Parinaud's syndrome
  - (ii) Argyll Robertson pupils
  - (iii) Holmes–Adie syndrome
  - (iv) aberrant nerve III regeneration
  - (v) diabetes mellitus
  - (vi) myotonic dystrophy

OPTIC DISC ABNORMALITIES

1 Congenital optic pit:
- (a) often inferotemporal and unilateral
- (b) associated with serous macular detachment
- (c) arcuate scotomata and other field defects occur

2 Optic disc coloboma:
- (a) deep excavation
- (b) may produce various field defects
- (c) vision normal or reduced

3 "Morning glory" syndrome:
- (a) unilateral dysplastic coloboma
- (b) cup filled with glial tissue
- (c) cup surrounded by pigment ring
- (d) spoke like radiation of vessels
- (e) poor vision
- (f) retinal detachment occurs

4 Tilted disc:
  (a) often bilateral
  (b) associated with:
      (i) high myopia
      (ii) astigmatism
      (iii) field defects
5 Optic nerve hypoplasia:
  (a) small disc with pale halo
  (b) poor vision
  (c) various field defects
  (d) relative afferent pupil defect if unilateral
  (e) associated with:
      (i) aniridia
      (ii) de Morsier's syndrome
      (iii) microphthalmos
6 Myelinated nerve fibres:
  (a) congenital
  (b) white flame shaped patches
  (c) usually adjacent to disc
  (d) enlarged blind spot
7 Melanocytoma:
  (a) benign melanotic disc lesion
  (b) often inferiorly
  (c) usually in dark skinned races
  (d) normal vision
8 Optic disc drusen:
  (a) congenital, often familial
  (b) 70% bilateral
  (c) absent optic cup
  (d) multiple opalescent bodies
  (e) autofluorescence
  (f) increasing prominence with age
  (g) associated with:
      (i) vitreous haemorrhage
      (ii) subretinal neovascular membranes
      (iii) angioid streaks
      (iv) retinitis pigmentosa
9 Bergmeister's papilla:
  (a) remnant of glial sheath of hyaloid artery
  (b) vision unaffected

CAUSES OF OPTIC DISC SWELLING

1 Papilloedema
2 Papillitis
3 Accelerated hypertension
4 Intraocular inflammation
5 Central retinal vein occlusion
6 Ischaemic optic neuropathy
7 Optic nerve compression

8 Infiltrative optic neuropathy, e.g. lymphoma
9 Ocular hypotony
10 Toxic optic neuropathy
11 Optic disc drusen and hypermetropia (pseudo-swelling)
12 Diabetic optic neuropathy (papillopathy)

Papilloedema

1 Features:
   (a) disc swelling in the presence of raised intracranial pressure
   (b) vision usually good until late stages
   (c) obscurations may occur
2 Stages:
   (a) early:
      (i) absent spontaneous venous pulsation
      (ii) nerve fibre swelling at disc
      (iii) disc capillary plexus dilatation
      (iv) peripapillary haemorrhage
      (v) retinal folds
   (b) acute decompensated:
      (i) grossly swollen hyperaemic disc
      (ii) masking of blood vessels
      (iii) loss of cup
      (iv) haemorrhages
      (v) cotton wool spots
   (c) chronic:
      (i) Champagne cork appearance
      (ii) fewer haemorrhages
      (iii) macular star
      (iv) arcuate field loss (late)
   (d) terminal:
      (i) pale atrophied flat disc
      (ii) arteriolar attenuation
      (iii) poor vision

Optic neuritis

1 Features:
   (a) reduced vision
   (b) paracentral or central scotoma
   (c) pain with ocular movement
   (d) colour desaturation
   (e) Uhthoff's phenomenon
   (f) Pulfrich's phenomenon
   (g) relative afferent pupillary defect
   (h) increased latency on VE: inflammatory optic neuritis only
2 Types:
   (a) papillitis:
      (i) disc swelling
      (ii) hyperaemia
      (iii) haemorrhages

(b) retrobulbar neuritis: normal disc
(c) neuroretinitis:
   (i) papillitis
   (ii) macular star
3 Causes:
   (a) multiple sclerosis (most common cause)
   (b) Devic's disease (neuromyelitis optica): affects children and young adults; rapid severe bilateral visual loss accompanied by paraplegia
   (c) viral encephalitis
   (d) infectious mononucleosis
   (e) herpes zoster ophthalmicus
   (f) contiguous inflammation of orbit, meninges, or sinuses
   (g) granulomatous inflammation of optic nerve, e.g. syphilis, TB, sarcoidosis
   (h) intraocular inflammation

Anterior ischaemic optic neuropathy (AION)

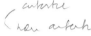

1 Causes:
   (a) giant cell arteritis
   (b) collagen vascular diseases
   (c) arteriosclerosis
   (d) systemic hypertension
   (e) systemic hypotension
   (f) carotid artery disease
   (g) diabetes mellitus

Diabetic papillopathy

1 Juvenile onset (type 1 diabetics)
2 Second to third decades
3 Bilateral involvement in 75%
4 Mild to moderate reduction in vision
5 Recovery in 6 months
6 Features: mild to florid disc swelling, macular oedema with exudates, and star formation.
7 Management: nothing specific apart from good diabetic control

Optic atrophy

1 Congenital or hereditary:
   (a) Leber's hereditary optic atrophy
   (b) dominant and recessive types
   (c) infantile optic atrophy
   (d) congenital syphilis
2 Secondary to raised intracranial pressure
3 Secondary to retinal disease (consecutive):
   (a) vascular, e.g. central retinal artery occlusion
   (b) inflammatory, e.g. Behçet's
   (c) choroiditis
   (d) retinitis pigmentosa

(e) glaucoma

4 Secondary to optic neuritis or neuropathy:
  (a) vascular, e.g. ischaemic optic neuropathy
  (b) multiple sclerosis
  (c) vitamin B_1 deficiency
  (d) toxic neuropathy, e.g. drugs, heavy metals
  (e) infection, e.g. syphilis

5 Secondary to optic nerve compression:
  (a) tumours, e.g. meningioma, pituitary adenoma
  (b) aneurysm
  (c) dysthyroid eye disease
  (d) infiltrative disease, e.g. sarcoid, lymphoma
  (e) infection, e.g. orbital cellulitis
  (f) bony overgrowth, e.g. Paget's disease

6 Secondary to trauma

7 Secondary to metabolic disease, e.g. mucopolysaccharidoses

CHIASMAL LESIONS

1 Pituitary tumours:
  (a) middle aged adults (M = F)
  (b) present with visual failure and/or hormonal imbalance
  (c) chromophobe most common (often prolactinoma)
  (d) chromophobe or basophil can secrete ACTH (Cushing's disease)
  (e) eosinophil can secrete growth hormone (gigantism or acromegaly)
  (f) 30% tumours non-functioning
  (g) bitemporal hemianopia and optic atrophy
  (h) late "hemifield slide phenomena" and post fixational blindness
  (i) large pituitary fossa, double floor sign, bony erosion on skull radiograph
  (j) treatment:
     (i) dopamine antagonists for prolactinoma and to a lesser extent acromegaly
     (ii) correct hormone deficiencies
     (iii) surgery (usually trans-sphenoidal)
     (iv) radiotherapy (larger adenomas) *postoperatively*

2 Meningioma:
  (a) adults (especially middle aged women)
  (b) present with visual failure
  (c) situated at sphenoidal ridge, tuberculum sella, olfactory groove
  (d) often asymmetrical field loss, e.g. junctional scotoma
  (e) optic atrophy
  (f) hyperostosis seen on skull radiograph
  (g) surgical treatment
  (h) good prognosis if complete excision

3 Craniopharyngioma:
  (a) children and young adults; M = F
  (b) present with features of raised intracranial pressure, hormonal imbalance, or visual failure

child — hypothalami / hypopit.
(adults — vit
mi diful
hypopit .

[handwritten left margin: ef involve 3rd vent.]

    (c) various patterns of field loss
    (d) papilloedema or optic atrophy
    (e) slow growing, often cystic
    (f) calcification shows on skull radiograph
    (g) surgical treatment
    (h) less good prognosis

4 Aneurysms: *supra Chiasmal int. Carotid*
    (a) middle aged adults; M = F
    (b) present with visual failure and/or ophthalmoplegia *(Cav. Sinus)*
    (c) internal carotid, anterior communicating, or ophthalmic arteries
    (d) field loss depends on position of lesion
    (e) calcification or bony erosion on skull radiograph
    (f) surgical treatment
    (g) variable prognosis
    (h) investigate with magnetic resonance angiography (MRA) or 4 vessel angiography

5 Optic nerve or glioma of chiasma:
    (a) children (80% are under 10)
    (b) 60% have von Recklinghausen's disease
    (c) present with visual loss
    (d) field loss depends on position of lesion
    (e) optic atrophy (occasional papilloedema)
    (f) very slow growing
    (g) enlarged optic foramen on skull radiograph
    (h) observe (occasional radiotherapy or surgery)

6 Other chiasmal lesions:
    (a) multiple sclerosis *(acute stage → ↑ Chiasma)*
    (b) trauma
    (c) basal meningitis or arachnoiditis *(sarcoid)*
    (d) sphenoidal sinus mucocele or carcinoma
    (e) pituitary infarction (apoplexy) *acute hge infarction of pit. adenoma*
    (f) empty sellar syndrome *sever headach, meningeal irritn + Chiasmal syndrome*

RETROCHIASMAL LESIONS

All have homonymous field defects; a complete homonymous hemianopia has no localising value. Lesions of optic tract and lateral geniculate body produce incongruous field loss. Visual acuity usually unaffected.

1 Optic tract lesions:
    (a) features:
        (i) rare
        (ii) incongruous hemianopic field loss
    (b) causes:
        (i) posteriorly extending chiasmal lesions
        (ii) vascular lesions

2 Temporal lobe lesions:
    (a) features:
        (i) affecting Meyer's loop
        (ii) causing upper homonymous quadrantanopia

(iii) if incongruous, denser on nasal side
(b) causes:
  (i) gliomas
  (ii) vascular lesions
  (iii) surgical trauma
3 Parietal lobe lesions:
(a) features:
  (i) complete homonymous hemianopia
  (ii) occasionally lower quadrantanopsia
  (iii) decreased optokinetic nystagmus towards side of lesion
  (iv) associated with apraxia
(b) causes:
  (i) metastases
  (ii) glioma
  (iii) meningioma
  (iv) middle cerebral artery thrombosis
4 Occipital lobe lesions:
(a) features:
  (i) congruous homonymous hemianopia
  (ii) may have macular sparing
(b) causes:
  (i) vascular (90%)
  (ii) tumours
  (iii) post-traumatic (*contre coup*)

NUCLEAR AND INFRANUCLEAR PALSIES

Oculomotor (III) nerve palsies
1 Features:
(a) may be complete, pupil sparing, or combined with sympathetic paralysis
(b) ptosis
(c) fixed dilated pupil (if complete)
(d) eye abducted and depressed
2 Nuclear lesions:
(a) vascular, demyelination
(b) usually incomplete
(c) unilateral nerve III palsy with contralateral superior rectus palsy
(d) bilateral with sparing of levator palpebrae superioris
3 Fascicular lesion:
(a) vascular, demyelination, or tumours
(b) Weber's syndrome (nerve III palsy and contralateral hemiparesis)
(c) Benedikt's syndrome (nerve III palsy and contralateral cerebellar signs)
4 Interpeduncular lesions:
(a) posterior communicating artery aneurysm
(b) painful and complete
(c) other causes: trauma, meningitis, raised intracranial pressure
5 Cavernous sinus lesions:

(a) aneurysm, thrombosis, fistula, extrasellar pituitary tumour
(b) often combined with palsies of nerves IV, V, VI
(c) may be paralysis of pupillary sympathetics

6 Superior orbital fissure, orbital apex, and orbital lesions:
   (a) tumours, granulomatous infiltrate, trauma, orbital cellulitis, dysthyroid eye disease
   (b) proptosis
   (c) may be combined with palsies of nerves IV, V, VI

7 Other causes of nerve III palsy:
   (a) diabetes mellitus (often pupil sparing)
   (b) arteriosclerosis
   (c) autoimmune vasculitis
   (d) herpes zoster ophthalmicus
   (e) migraine

8 Aberrant nerve III regeneration:
   (a) several patterns
   (b) lid elevation on downgaze or adduction
   (c) adduction or retraction on downgaze or upgaze
   (d) various ocular movements producing miosis

Trochlear (IV) nerve palsies

1 Features:
   (a) oblique diplopia, worse on downgaze
   (b) hypertropia (greater for near)
   (c) head tilt and face turn to opposite side with chin down
   (d) most common causes are trauma and vascular (hypertension, diabetes)

2 Bielschowsky's test: hypertropia on tilting head to side of lesion

3 Types:
   (a) isolated: unilateral or bilateral (usually traumatic)
   (b) associated with other palsies
   (c) complicated: dorsal midbrain lesions

Abducent (VI) nerve palsies

1 Features:
   (a) horizontal diplopia (greater for distance)
   (b) complete or partial failure of abduction
   (c) face turn towards affected side
   (d) esotropia

2 Types:
   (a) isolated, e.g. vascular raised intracranial pressure
   (b) associated with other palsies, cavernous sinus disease
   (c) complicated:
       (i) Millard–Gubler syndrome—VI, VII, and contralateral hemiparesis—pontine lesion
       (ii) Toville's syndrome—V, VI, VII, VIII, and Hofner's syndrome
       (iii) Gradenigo's syndrome—VI with otitis media caused by periostitis of petrous bone

Aetiology of ocular nerve palsies
1 Idiopathic (25%)
2 Infarction (III, VI): diabetes mellitus, hypertension
3 Trauma (IV)
4 Pressure from aneurysm (III)
5 Multiple sclerosis (VI, III)
6 Pressure from neoplasia
7 Tentorial herniation (III)
8 Inflammations:
  (a) basal meningitis
  (b) herpes zoster ophthalmicus
  (c) vasculitis
  (d) sarcoidosis
  (e) acute infections
  (f) polyneuropathy
9 Raised intracranial pressure (III, VI)
10 Caroticocavernous fistulae (multiple palsies)
11 Ophthalmoplegic migraine
12 Congenital

HORIZONTAL GAZE PALSIES

Supranuclear
1 Congenital oculomotor apraxia:
  (a) bilateral saccadic paralysis
  (b) associated with head thrusting
2 Möbius' syndrome:
  (a) horizontal gaze palsy
  (b) palsies of nerve VI, VII
  (c) occasionally palsies of nerve IX, XII
3 Focal frontal lesions: contralateral saccadic palsy
4 Focal parieto-occipital lesions: ipsilateral pursuit palsy ("cog wheel" pursuit)—decreased optokinetic nystagmus towards side of lesion
5 Focal tegmental lesion: ipsilateral pursuit and saccadic palsy
6 Focal pontine lesion (PPRF): ipsilateral horizontal gaze palsy
7 Diffuse lesions:
  (a) Parkinson's disease
  (b) Huntington's disease
8 Metabolic lesions:
  (a) hyperglycaemia
  (b) Wernicke's encephalopathy
  (c) Wilson's disease
9 Drug induced:
  (a) tricyclic antidepressants
  (b) phenytoin
  (c) phenothiazines
10 Pseudogaze palsies:
  (a) myasthenia gravis
  (b) chronic progressive external ophthalmoplegia

Internuclear ophthalmoplegia

1 Features:
  (a) lesion in medial longitudinal fasciculus
  (b) limitation of adduction of one eye
  (c) ataxic nystagmus in abducting eye
  (d) unilateral or bilateral
  (e) symmetrical or asymmetrical
  (f) convergence usually good
  (g) diplopia not always present
2 Causes:
  (a) multiple sclerosis
  (b) arteriosclerosis
  (c) tumours (gliomas)

"One and a half" syndrome

1 Features:
  (a) unilateral pontine lesion
  (b) affects horizontal gaze centre and medial longitudinal fasciculus
  (c) ipsilateral gaze palsy and internuclear ophthalmoplegia
  (d) only movement is abduction of contralateral eye (with ataxic nystagmus)
2 Causes:
  (a) multiple sclerosis
  (b) basilar artery occlusion
  (c) pontine metastasis

VERTICAL GAZE PALSIES

1 Focal midbrain disease, e.g. Parinaud's syndrome
2 Basal ganglion disease, e.g. Steele–Richardson syndrome, kernicterus
3 Metabolic disease, e.g. maple syrup disease, Wernicke's encephalopathy
4 Drug induced
5 Pseudogaze palsies

OCULAR MANIFESTATIONS OF BASAL GANGLIA DISEASE

1 Parkinson's disease:
  (a) seborrhoeic blepharitis
  (b) reduced blinking
  (c) reduced saccades (hypometric)
  (d) reduced glabellar reflex suppression
  (e) blepharospasm
  (f) oculogyric crisis (especially drug induced)
2 Steele–Richardson syndrome (progressive supranuclear palsy):
  (a) decreased saccades (horizontal early, later vertical)
  (b) progressive vertical and horizontal gaze palsy
  (c) spasm of fixation

    (d) retention of pursuit/doll's head movements
3 Wilson's disease:
    (a) sunflower cataract
    (b) Kayser–Fleischer ring in Descemet's membrane
    (c) various ocular motor defects (nystagmus, upgaze paresis, slow saccades)
4 Kernicterus: progressive loss of eye movement especially upgaze

HEADACHE AND FACIAL PAIN

1 Acute:
    (a) subarachnoid haemorrhage
    (b) meningitis/encephalitis
    (c) focal inflammation of scalp
    (d) sinusitis
    (e) dental infection
    (f) acute uveitis
    (g) acute glaucoma
    (h) scleritis
    (i) herpes zoster
    (j) cervical spondylitis
    (k) giant cell arteritis
    (l) trauma
2 Recurrent:
    (a) migraine
    (b) cluster headaches
    (c) asthenopia
    (d) cerebral aneurysm or angioma
    (e) hypertensive headache (severe hypertension)
3 Chronic:
    (a) muscle tension
    (b) depression
    (c) cerebral tumour
    (d) pituitary or nasopharyngeal tumour
    (e) Paget's disease
    (f) post-traumatic
    (g) raised intracranial pressure
    (h) chronic subdural haemorrhage
    (i) postherpetic neuralgia
    (j) trigeminal neuralgia
    (k) Costen's syndrome (temporomandibular osteoarthritis)

MIGRAINE

1 Common migraine:
    (a) any age; M = F
    (b) little or no prodrome
    (c) throbbing headache
    (d) photophobia

    (e) nausea
    (f) seeks seclusion
    (g) pallor
2 Classic migraine:
    (a) any age; M = F
    (b) less severe when older
    (c) trigger factors
    (d) visual prodrome, e.g. fortification spectra
    (e) intense headache (unilateral)
    (f) photophobia
    (g) nausea
    (h) seeks seclusion
    (i) pallor
3 Complicated migraines:
    (a) hemiplegic or hemiparetic
    (b) ophthalmoplegic
    (c) retinal
    (d) basilar
    (e) abdominal
    (f) oculosympathetic
4 Childhood migraine:
    (a) brief attacks
    (b) pallor, nausea, vomiting
    (c) usually no headaches

NYSTAGMUS

Defect of ocular posture control.
1 Types:
    (a) 1: pendular (associated with poor vision)
    (b) 2: jerk (associated with CNS disease)
    (c) 3: horizontal or vertical
    (d) 4: oblique
    (e) 5: rotary
    (f) 6: fixed
2 Alternatively:
    (a) physiological:
        (i) optokinetic
        (ii) vestibular
        (iii) endpoint
    (b) vestibular:
        (i) lesion in inner ear, nerve VIII, brainstem/vestibular pathways
        (ii) jerk, present in primary position of gaze but usually lessens on fixation
        (iii) can have associated vertigo
    (c) gaze evoked:
        (i) jerk, not present in primary position of gaze
        (ii) main causes—drugs (anticonvulsants, major tranquillisers)
        (iii) brainstem/cerebellar lesions
    (d) motor imbalance:

    (i) congenital nystagmus:
- pendular or jerk
- X-linked or autosomal dominant
- binocular, usually horizontal
- damps with convergence
- may nod or have compensatory head posture for null point
- astigmatism common
- vision 6/12 to 6/36, better near vision

    (ii) latent nystagmus—in dissociated vertical deviation.

    (iii) ataxic nystagmus—in internuclear ophthalmoplegia

    (iv) spasmus nutans:
- infantile pendular nystagmus
- compensatory head posture and head nodding
- resolves by the age of 3

    (v) periodic alternating nystagmus—in brainstem disease (usually disseminated sclerosis or vascular)

    (vi) downbeat nystagmus—foramen magnum lesions

    (vii) upbeat nystagmus:
- drug toxicity, e.g. anticonvulsants
- posterior fossa lesions

    (viii) convergence–retraction nystagmus—in dorsal midbrain syndrome, e.g. Parinaud's syndrome

    (ix) see-saw nystagmus—chiasmal lesions

(e) sensory deprivation:

    (i) pendular

    (ii) causes:
- congenital or early onset cataracts
- macular or optic nerve hypoplasia
- albinism
- Leber's congenital amaurosis
- congenital glaucoma

Causes of external ophthalmoplegia

1 Palsies of nerves III, IV, VI
2 Thyroid ophthalmopathy
3 Orbital trauma
4 Orbital tumour
5 Orbital cellulitis
6 Myopathies
7 Myasthenia gravis
8 Special oculomotility syndromes, e.g. Duane's syndrome
9 Myositis
10 Gaze palsies

Myasthenia gravis

1 Features:
    (a) autoimmune abnormality at neuromuscular junctions
    (b) antiacetylcholine receptor antibodies (IgG)
    (c) F > M

    (d) average age of onset 15–50 years
    (e) 75% present with ocular features
    (f) increasing fatiguability on exercise
    (g) variable muscle weakness
    (h) dysarthria, dysphagia
    (i) facial weakness ("snarl")
    (j) respiratory failure
    (k) variable ptosis
    (l) variable ophthalmoplegia

2 Associations:
    (a) penicillamine treatment
    (b) rheumatoid arthritis
    (c) systemic lupus erythematosus
    (d) thyrotoxicosis
    (e) thymic hyperplasia or tumour

3 Treatment:
    (a) anticholinesterases
    (b) steroids
    (c) thymectomy
    (d) plasmapheresis
    (e) immunosuppressive drugs
    (f) conservative ocular treatment, e.g. ptosis crutches

16
MEDICAL OPHTHALMOLOGY

ARTHRITIDES AND CONNECTIVE TISSUE DISEASES

Rheumatoid arthritis

A chronic systemic inflammatory condition characterised by a persistent, peripheral, symmetrical polyarthritis; common disease. F > M. *unsure*
1 General features:
  (a) arthritis: symmetrical and predominately peripheral
  (b) nodules: on pressure points, tendons, and internal organs
  (c) vascular:
    (i) Raynaud's phenomenon
    (ii) splinter haemorrhages in nailfolds
    (iii) necrotising arteritis affecting digits and occasionally internal organs
    (iv) skin ulceration
    (v) occasionally organ infarction
  (d) lung: nodules and fibrosis
  (e) heart: pericarditis
  (f) neuromuscular:
    (i) proximal myopathy and sensory neuropathy
    (ii) atlantoaxial subluxation may result in spinal cord compression
  (g) kidneys: amyloidosis
2 Ocular features:
  (a) keratoconjunctivitis sicca
  (b) cornea:
    (i) keratitis
    (ii) peripheral corneal thinning ("contact lens" cornea); if very severe may perforate
  (c) episcleritis
  (d) scleritis

Systemic lupus erythematosus

Multisystem autoimmune condition characterised by autoantibodies to double stranded DNA. F > M.

1 General features:
   (a) joints: <u>migratory</u> symmetrical <u>polyarthralgia</u>   *non-erosive*
   (b) skin:
      (i) facial butterfly rash
      (ii) photosensitivity *rash*
      (iii) discoid rash
      (iv) nailfold infarcts
      ✳(v) Raynaud's phenomenon
   (c) kidneys: antigen–antibody complex deposition which may result in proteinuria, nephritic syndrome, or chronic renal failure with hypertension
   (d) lungs: pleurisy
   (e) heart: pericarditis
   (f) nervous system:
      (i) peripheral neuropathy
      (ii) psychosis
2 Ocular features:
   (a) eyelid erythema with facial butterfly rash
   (b) telangiectasia *conj.*
   (c) keratoconjunctivitis sicca
   (d) keratitis with peripheral corneal thinning *? 2° to scleritis*
   ✳(e) scleritis *+ uveitis*
   (f) retinopathy:
      (i) "<u>primary</u>"—<u>retinal vasculitis</u> with cotton wool spots; disc oedema and haemorrhages
      (ii) "<u>secondary</u>" <u>to hypertension</u>

Scleroderma

Chronic disease dominated by cutaneous manifestations. F > M.
1 General features:
   (a) skin:
      ✳(i) Raynaud's phenomenon
      (ii) tight skin with swelling in early stages
      (iii) "purse string mouth"
      (iv) nailfold infarcts
      (v) calcinosis
   (b) bowel: oesophageal and small intestine fibrosis, causing dysphagia and malabsorption
   (c) lungs: fibrosis
   (d) heart: myocarditis and pericarditis
   (e) kidneys: hypertension and renal failure
   (f) musculoskeletal: polyarthralgia and myositis
2 Ocular features:
   (a) tight skin over eyelids causing punctal ectropion and epiphora
   (b) lagophthalmos
   (c) keratoconjunctivitis sicca

(d) iris changes suggestive of atrophy
(e) retinopathy usually caused by renal hypertension

Polymyositis and dermatomyositis

Rare; F > M.
1 General features:
  (a) muscular system:
      (i) girdle weakness (shoulder and hip)
      (ii) muscle pain and weakness
      (iii) dysphagia and dysphonia from laryngeal and pharyngeal muscle involvement
  (b) skin:
      (i) purple "heliotrope" rash
      (ii) violet oedematous lesions over small joints of hands
      (iii) nailfold infarcts
      (iv) telangiectasia
      (v) Raynaud's phenomena
  (c) joints: transient arthralgia
  (d) heart: cardiomyopathy
  (e) lungs: fibrosis
2 Ocular features:
  (a) a heliotrope (purple) rash over the eyelids
  (b) periorbital oedema
  (c) retinopathy with cotton wool spots
  (d) diplopia resulting from ocular myopathy

Sjögren's syndrome

Chronic inflammatory autoimmune disorder characterised by a mixed cellular infiltration of exocrine glands, notably the lacrimal and salivary glands.
1 Features:
  (a) dry eyes (xerophthalmia)
  (b) dry mouth (xerostomia)
  (c) dyspareunia and chest infections
2 Types:
  (a) primary Sjögren's syndrome:
      (i) the "sicca" complex with no associated disease
      (ii) hypergammaglobulinaemia 50%
      (iii) rheumatoid factor 80%
      (iv) anti-nuclear factor 80%
      (v) other autoantibodies (salivary gland, gastric parietal cell, and smooth muscle)
      (vi) cryoglobulinaemia
  (b) secondary Sjögren's syndrome: associated with a connective tissue disease
3 Associations:
  (a) rheumatoid arthritis
  (b) systemic lupus erythematosus
  (c) polymyositis/dermatomyositis

    (d) scleroderma
    (e) polyarteritis nodosa
    (f) Graves' disease
    (g) chronic active hepatitis and primary biliary cirrhosis
    (h) myasthenia gravis
    (i) coeliac disease
    (j) mixed connective tissue disease
    (k) non-Hodgkin's lymphoma; risk increased 40 times in Sjögren's syndrome
4 Pathology: inflammation and infiltration by plasma cells and lymphocytes with subsequent fibrosis
5 Management:
    (a) treat associated conditions
    (b) tear replacement
    (c) topical mucolytic agent
    (d) vaginal lubricants

VASCULITIDES

Giant cell arteritis
Arteritis affecting medium and large muscular arteries. Patients rarely less than 60 years old. F > M.
1 General features:
    (a) fever, malaise, anorexia, and weight loss
    (b) headaches
    (c) tender temporal or other superficial cranial arteries; scalp ulceration may occur
    (d) jaw claudication or pain in tongue on eating
    (e) arteritis:
        (i) aortitis
        (ii) bowel infarction
        (iii) myocardial infarction
        (iv) cerebral infarction
    (f) musculoskeletal: muscle weakness and pain; arthralgia
    (g) polymyalgia rheumatica syndrome: main feature is proximal limb girdle weakness and pain
    (h) ESR usually high (but not in 30s)
2 Ocular features:
    (a) ischaemic optic neuropathy as a result of occlusion of posterior ciliary arteries
    (b) less commonly, central retinal artery occlusion
    (c) ocular palsies-caused by muscle or nerve ischaemia
    (d) cortical blindness
    (e) anterior segment ischaemia
3 Histology:
    (a) artery wall thickened by inflammatory cells (histiocytes, lymphocytes, and giant cells, fibrinoid necrosis); skip lesions
    (b) reaction directed against medial muscle cells and internal elastic lamina

(c) vascular lumen narrowed by fibroblastic proliferation in lumen; may be occluded by thrombus

Polyarteritis nodosa

Systemic vasculitis affecting medium sized and small arteries. M > F.
1 General features:
   (a) kidney:
      (i) hypertension which may be malignant
      (ii) nephritic or nephrotic syndrome
      (iii) renal failure
   (b) heart:
      (i) myocardial infarction
      (ii) angina
      (iii) pericarditis
   (c) bowel: pain and infarction
   (d) skin: arteritic lesions
   (e) joints: arthritis
   (f) nervous system: peripheral neuropathy
2 Ocular features:
   (a) necrotising sclerokeratitis
   (b) retinopathy:
      (i) "primary" vasculitis with occlusion
      (ii) "secondary" due to hypertension
   (c) yellow choroidal foci *Choroidal vasculitis*
   (d) ischaemic optic neuropathy
   (e) transient focal detachments
   (f) rarely aneurysms of retinal vessels

Wegener's granulomatosis

1 General features:
   (a) necrotising vasculitis with involvement of:
      (i) upper respiratory tract—haemoptysis
      (ii) kidneys (renal failure major cause of death)
      (iii) skin lesions
      (iv) middle ear and sinus lesions
      (v) serum antineutrophil cytoplasmic antibodies (ANCA) may be diagnostic
   (b) in addition pyrexia, weight loss, peripheral neuropathy, and cerebral vasculitis
2 Ocular features:
   (a) non-specific conjunctivitis with subconjunctival haemorrhages
   (b) episcleritis
   (c) scleritis *necrotizing scleritis*
   (d) corneal infiltration and ulceration *Periph-ulcerative keratitis*
   (e) nasolacrimal duct obstruction
   (f) orbital involvement: proptosis, painful ophthalmoplegia, chemosis, retinal venous congestion, and optic nerve involvement
   (g) retinopathy: arterial narrowing, venous tortuosity, cotton wool

orbital vasculitis - proptosis
from
NLD)
scleritis - necrotizing scleritis, uveitis, P ulcerative keratitis
retinal vasculitis.

spots, choroidal thickening, cystoid macular oedema, and choroidoretinitis

AIDS (ACQUIRED IMMUNE DEFICIENCY SYNDROME)

1 Definition: the diagnosis is made in people who have both:
   (a) a reliably diagnosed disease that is at least moderately indicative of underlying cellular immune deficiency, e.g. Kaposi's sarcoma, *Pneumocystis carinii* pneumonia, or cytomegalovirus retinitis
   (b) no other known underlying cause of cellular immune deficiency
2 Causal agent: human immunodeficiency virus (HIV); was also known as human T cell lymphotropic virus (HTLV-III) and lymphadenopathy associated virus (LAV)
3 Clinical states after HIV infection:
   (a) acquired immune deficiency syndrome
   (b) aids related complex (ARC): people with 2 or more symptoms or signs of specific, chronic, unexplained conditions for 3 months or longer, together with 2 or more abnormal laboratory values:
       (i) signs and symptoms—pyrexia of more than 2 months, chronic diarrhoea, weight loss of 10% body weight, malaise and lethargy, persistent generalised lymphadenopathy, hepatosplenomegaly, hairy leukoplakia, or minor oral infections
       (ii) laboratory findings—HIV antibodies or virus isolation, lymphopenia, leukopenia, anaemia, thrombocytopenia, raised ESR, cholesterol, immunoglobulins, or immunological abnormalities
   (c) persistent generalised lymphadenopathy (PGL): unexplained lymphadenopathy in at least 2 extrainguinal sites for more than 3 months
   (d) asymptomatic carriers of the virus
4 Prognosis:
   (a) AIDS is universally fatal; life expectancy depends on presenting disease, e.g. Kaposi's sarcoma alone carries a mean survival of 125 weeks as opposed to *Pneumocystis carinii* where mean survival is 35 weeks
   (b) 60% of infected individuals remain asymptomatic carriers, 33% develop PGL or ARC, and the remaining 7% develop AIDS within 3 years
5 Transmission (UK, 1986):
   (a) homosexuals/bisexuals (89%)
   (b) recipients of blood products (5·5%)
   (c) association with Africa (3%)
   (d) intravenous drug users (1%)
   (e) heterosexual contacts (1%)
   (f) unknown (0·5%)
6 General features:
   (a) pulmonary:
       (i) infectious—*Pneumocystis carinii*, cytomegalovirus, *Mycobacterium avium*, *Cryptococcus neoformans*, *Mycobacterium*

tuberculosis
- (ii) non-infectious—non-specific pneumonitis, adult respiratory distress syndrome
- (b) skin:
  - (i) infectious—herpes zoster and simplex, warts, candidiasis and other fungal infections, Kaposi's sarcoma
  - (ii) non-infectious—immune complex vasculitis, thrombocytopenic purpura, hairy leukoplakia, and seborrhoeic dermatitis
- (c) gastrointestinal: Kaposi's sarcoma, cytomegalovirus, *Cryptosporidium* spp., shigellosis, salmonellosis, *Campylobacter* spp., *Entamoeba histolytica*, *Giardia lamblia*, candidiasis, herpes simplex
- (d) CNS:
  - (i) cytomegalovirus—meningoencephalitis
  - (ii) *Toxoplasma gondii*—mass lesions
  - (iii) *Cryptococcus neoformans*—relapsing subacute meningitis
  - (iv) CNS lymphomas—mass lesions
  - (v) Papovaviruses—diffuse subacute brain disease
  - (vi) herpes simplex virus—encephalomyelitis
  - (vii) HIV encephalopathy—progressive dementia

7 Ocular features:
- (a) conjunctival Kaposi's sarcoma
- (b) keratitis
- (c) episcleritis
- (d) uveitis
- (e) retinal oedema and haemorrhages
- (f) cotton wool spots (even those occurring on their own) indicate a poor prognosis)
- (g) flame shaped haemorrhages
- (h) retinal vascular sheathing
- (i) choroidal granulomata
- (j) secondary cytomegalovirus retinitis; CMV features, i.e.:
  - (i) unifocal or multifocal "pizza pie" retinopathy
  - (ii) necrotising retinitis
  - (iii) retinal vasculitides
  - (iv) retinal detachments
- (k) papillitis
- (l) increased length of eyelashes *trichomegaly.*

INFECTIOUS MONONUCLEOSIS (GLANDULAR FEVER)

Caused by the Epstein–Barr virus.
1 General features:
- (a) fever and malaise
- (b) pharyngitis with palatal petechiae and tonsillar exudate
- (c) cervical lymphadenopathy and hepatosplenomegaly
- (d) arthralgia
- (e) maculopapular rash (especially if ampicillin given)
2 Ocular features:
- (a) oedema of eyelids and periorbital tissues

    (b) conjunctivitis (follicular or membranous)
    (c) subconjunctival haemorrhages

BLOOD DISORDERS

Ocular features of any anaemia

1 Pale conjunctiva
2 Retinal haemorrhages
3 Retinal haemorrhages with white centres (Roth's spots)
4 Dilated retinal veins

Causes of Roth's spots

1 Anaemia
2 Subacute bacterial endocarditis
3 Leukaemia
4 Hypertension
5 Diabetes

Leukaemias
1 Ocular features (eye may be involved at presentation, or as a site of disease recurrence):
    (a) orbital involvement (one of the more common causes of proptosis in children)
    (b) lid haemorrhage
    (c) iris involvement with hypopyon or hyphaema
    (d) vitreous infiltration (rare)
    (e) retinal neovascularisation
    (f) leukaemic retinopathy with retinal haemorrhages, Roth's spots, and tortuous dilated veins
    (g) cotton wool spots
    (h) optic nerve head infiltration
    (i) papilloedema resulting from raised intracranial pressure from CNS infiltration

Myeloma

1 Ocular features:
    (a) corneal crystalline deposits
    (b) conjunctival vessel sludging
    (c) retinal vascular tortuosity and haemorrhages
    (d) "sausage link" retinal veins, particularly in Waldenström's macro-globulinaemia (IgM myeloma)
    (e) cotton wool spots
    (f) uveal effusion
    (g) optic disc swelling

SKIN DISORDERS

Pseudoxanthoma elasticum (PXE)

Autosomal recessive.

1 General features:
   (a) skin changes on neck, axilla, antecubital fossa, and paraumbilical region ("chicken skin")
   (b) vascular:
      (i) weak pulses
      (ii) calcification
      (iii) intermittent claudication
      (iv) angina
   (c) gastrointestinal: bleeding
2 Ocular features:
   (a) angioid streaks and PXE = Grönblad–Strandberg syndrome
   (b) pigmentary retinal mottling (*peau d'orange*)
   (c) peripapillary choroidal atrophy
   (d) drusen at the optic nerve head

Atopic eczema

1 Ocular features:
   (a) chronic keratoconjunctivitis
   (b) keratoconus
   (c) giant papillary conjunctivitis
   (d) cataracts

Rosacea

1 General features:
   (a) telangiectasia, pustules, and papules
   (b) hypertrophic sebaceous glands
   (c) rhinophyma
   (d) 4th to 6th decades
2 Ocular features:
   (a) keratitis with peripheral vascularisation and thinning of the cornea; occasionally thinned areas may perforate; scarring and pannus may obscure vision
   (b) blepharoconjunctivitis
   (c) recurrent chalazia
   (d) episcleritis

PHAKOMATOSES

A group of disorders in which neurological abnormalities are combined with congenital defects of skin, retina, and other organs.

Sturge–Weber syndrome

Not inherited.

1 Features:
   (a) cutaneous angioma over the first and second divisions of trigeminal nerve

235

Ataxia telangiectasia (AR) — oculocut. teling. face, ear, flex. creas conj.
— Cerebellar telangiectasia → ataxia

② (b) associated meningeal angioma which may cause focal epilepsy; intracranial calcification of the angioma may occur — following the contour of the cortex gyri.

③ ocular { (c) glaucoma in 50% → ipsilat. buphthalmos.
{ (d) cavernous haemangioma of the choroid — if elevated → serous RD. Rx laser.

Iris — heterochromia + ang ipsilat.

Neurofibromatosis

Autosomal dominant; prevalence: at least 1 in 5000 population. *3520*

1 General features:
   (a) *café au lait* spots:
      (i) in children: >6 *café au lait* spots >0·5 cm in diameter
      (ii) in adults: >6 *café au lait* spots >1·5 cm in diameter — *at puberty ↑ with preg*
   (b) cutaneous neurofibromas *fibroma mulluscom over the body*
   ✱(c) axillary freckling (unique to neurofibromatosis)
   (d) 25% have neurological complications including:
      (i) plexiform neuromas
      (ii) tumours of the central nervous system — *brain, cord, periph nerv. sympathetic nerves*
      (iii) mental handicap
      (iv) epilepsy
   (e) congenital bone defects
   (f) endocrine tumours, e.g. phaeochromocytoma ✱*facial hemiatrophy*
   (g) scoliosis *(acquired)*

2 Ocular features:
   (a) eyelid plexiform neuroma *S shaped*
   Sit on iris — (b) iris nodules (Lisch nodules) (95%); confirms diagnosis if *café au lait* spots are also present *(Bil Iris melanocytic hamartoma)*
   (c) prominent corneal nerves (6%)
   (d) glaucoma *usually unilat + ipsilat. lid lesion, cong.*
   (e) choroidal naevi
   (f) astrocytic hamartomas (29%) *multiple small pale plaques*
   When bilat pathognomonic — (g) optic nerve gliomas and orbital tumours; also glial tissue overlying optic disc *15%. Chiasm, prolif. perineural rather than intraneural in isolated glioma, age...*
   Other orbit tumor ✱ meningioma of optic nerve or sphenoid — (h) spheno-orbital encephalocele (pulsatile proptosis) *cong defect in sphenoid { proptosis or enophth.*

3 Types:
   (a) type I: NF1; von Recklinghausen's (peripheral) neurofibromatosis (90%); major defining features are multiple *café au lait* spots, peripheral neurofibromas, and Lisch nodules; 30% develop one or more complications *Chrom 17*
   Chrom 22 — (b) type II: NF2; (bilateral) acoustic (central) neurofibromatosis; main features are bilateral acoustic neuromas and other nervous system tumours, particularly meningiomas *multiple, optic sheath + glioma. Juvenile PSC, retina + RPE hamartoma, larger cafe au lait spots*

Tuberous sclerosis

Autosomal dominant; 50% new mutations; defect located on chromosome 9 or 16.

1 General features:
   (a) mental handicap } West's syndrome
   (b) epilepsy
   (c) CNS hamartomas
   (d) adenoma sebaceum — *face, butterfly area age 2–5 pathognomonic*

✱ *Wyburn-mason* — retinal arterio venous malformation, divi → pup
Cong not inherited. — intracranial A-V.

(e) hypopigmented patches (ash leaf patches), more prominent under ultraviolet light

(f) *café au lait* spots

(g) shagreen patches on skin (fibrous thickenings)

(h) subungual fibromas *panangual, around nailbed* Pathognomic

(i) cardiac rhabdomyoma *80% of tuberous sclerosis*

2 Ocular features:

(a) hypopigmented iris spots *raised. Post pole*

(b) retinal hamartomas 50% ("mulberry" tumours when calcified) *flav. mulberry*

(c) papilloedema secondary to gliomas *+ ↑ICP.*

(d) nerve VI palsy secondary to raised intracranial pressure

(e) punched out depigmented retinal patches

Von Hippel–Lindau syndrome
ocular – angioma
Cap.

Autosomal dominant. *Chrom 3*

post fossa tumor – heangioblastoma.

1 General features:

(a) haemangioblastomas of: *Visceral – Renal < vas, hypnephron / Phaeochromocytoma*

   (i) cerebellum ⎤ with or

   (ii) medulla ⎟ without   *Clinical < Intracranial pres- / Hypertensive / retinopathy*

   (iii) pons ⎬ secondary

   (iv) spinal cord ⎦ polycythaemia

(b) visceral cysts *pancreas, epididymis*

(c) phaeochromocytoma *– check for ↑BP + vanillylmandelic acid*

(d) hypernephroma

2 Ocular features (50%):

(a) retinal and disc angiomas

(b) vitreous haemorrhage

(c) hard exudates when angioma leaks

(d) hypertensive retinopathy if associated with phaeochromocytoma

(e) papilloedema in presence of raised intracranial pressure

MISCELLANEOUS CONDITIONS

⎰ trisomy – non dysjunction ⎱
⎱ translocation < mutation / familial

Down's syndrome

Caused by trisomy or translocation of chromosome 21; 1/800 live births.

1 General features:

(a) short stature

(b) poorly developed bridge of nose

(c) enlarged, fissured tongue

(d) short fingers, curved inward (clinodactyly)

(e) broad hands with single palmar crease *(Siamese crease)*

(f) heart lesions (septal defects)

2 Ocular features:

(a) hypertelorism

(b) epicanthic folds with Mongoloid slant of eyelids

(c) ectropion

(d) blepharoconjunctivitis

(e) strabismus and nystagmus

(f) keratoconus sometimes presenting with acute hydrops

susceptibility to the effect of atropine

(g) Brushfield's spots on iris
(h) cataracts
(i) abnormal retinal hypoplastic disc *? optic atrophy .*
(j) refractive errors (mostly myopic) *+ astigmatism .*
Long glaucoma can occur .

Wilson's disease

Disease characterised by the widespread deposition of copper in tissues in association with a deficiency of ceruloplasmin (the α_2-globulin that binds most of the serum copper).

1 General features:
  (a) CNS (40%):
    (i) flapping tremor of wrists and shoulders
    (ii) mental changes
    (iii) spasticity, dysarthria, and dysphagia
  (b) hepatic (40%, < 10 years of age):
    (i) hepatosplenomegaly and jaundice
    (ii) cirrhosis and associated signs and symptoms
2 Ocular features:
  (a) Kayser–Fleischer ring: greenish-brown ring at level of Descemet's membrane
  (b) "sunflower cataract": central green lens opacity with tapering extensions

Gout

Clinical manifestation of sustained hyperuricaemia. M > F.
1 General features:
  (a) inflammation in a joint (classically metatarsophalangeal joint of big toe but may affect other joints)
  (b) tophi within joints, pinnae, and Achilles tendon
2 Ocular features:
  (a) conjunctivitis
  (b) episcleritis
  (c) scleritis
  (d) band keratopathy
  (e) urate deposits in cornea, sclera, lens, tarsus, and extraocular muscle tendons

Hyperlipidaemia

Conditions associated with raised levels of plasma cholesterol and triglyceride.
1 Causes:
  (a) primary, e.g. familial hypercholesterolaemia
  (b) secondary, e.g. diabetes mellitus, excess alcohol intake, and hypothyroidism
2 General features:
  (a) xanthomas:
    (i) extensor tendons (hands)
    (ii) Achilles tendons

  (iii) patellar tendons
  (iv) palmar
   (v) eruptive
(b) accelerated vascular disease:
   (i) angina
   (ii) myocardial infarction
  (iii) intermittent claudication
(c) pancreatitis and abdominal pain (hypertriglyceridaemia)
3 Ocular features:
(a) xanthelasmas
(b) arcus
(c) lipaemia retinalis

Osteogenesis imperfecta

1 General features:
(a) skeletal:
   (i) fragile bones which fracture easily
   (ii) short and often deformed extremities
  (iii) chest and skull deformities
(b) ears: hearing impairment from otosclerosis
(c) joints: flexible, tendons may rupture
(d) skin: thin, easily bruised
(e) heart: mitral and aortic valve prolapse
2 Ocular features:
(a) blue sclera
(b) keratoconus, megalocornea
(c) cataracts
(d) "Saturn ring": whitening of perilimbal sclera as a result of lack of
    pigmented uvea behind sclera

see page 90 HLA

Table 16.1 Some diseases associated with particular HLA types

HLA	Diseases	Relative risk (normal population = 1) (%)
HLA-A29	Birdshot choroidoretinopathy	97
HLA-B27	Ankylosing spondylitis	90
HLA-B27	Non-specific urethritis with arthritis	25
HLA-B27	Acute anterior uveitis	13
HLA-B27	Psoriatic arthritis	4
HLA-B5	Behçet's disease	6
HLA-B7 or -DR2	Multiple sclerosis	4
HLA-DW6	Psoriasis	13
HLA-DR3	Sjögren's disease	19
HLA-DR3	Systemic lupus erythematosus	6
HLA-DR3	Graves' disease	5
HLA-DR3	Juvenile onset diabetes mellitus	4
HLA-DR3	Myasthenia gravis	3
HLA-DR4	Juvenile onset diabetes mellitus	4
HLA-DR4	Rheumatoid arthritis	4

17
PHARMACOLOGY

METHODS OF DELIVERING OCULAR TREATMENT

1 Drops:
   (a) achieve a high concentration
   (b) quickly washed away; after 5 min >80% has entered the lacrimal drainage system
   (c) convenient for daytime use as cause minimal blurring of vision
   (d) preservatives, e.g. benzylalkonium chloride and thiomersal, can cause allergic reactions
2 Ointment:
   (a) longer contact time
   (b) lower drug concentration in tears
   (c) longer shelf life than drops
   (d) causes blurring of vision
3 Gels:
   (a) prolong contact time
   (b) newer gels may cause less blurring than ointment
4 Soft contact lenses:
   (a) absorb drugs (small molecules) when soaked in drug
   (b) deliver high concentrations over about 4 hours; note that normal soft lenses also absorb drugs
5 Membrane delivery:
   (a) relatively constant rate of drug delivery reducing side effects, e.g. Ocuserts resulting in less accommodative spasm and less fluctuation in intraocular pressure
   (b) deliver drug over a longer period
   (c) useful for patients with poor compliance, but easily lost
6 Subconjunctival/sub-Tenon's/orbital floor:
   (a) achieves high local concentration
   (b) can be painful, particularly with antibiotics; adequate oral analgesia and topical anaesthesia must be used
   (c) may cause scarring
7 Systemic: ocular penetration variable

Factors affecting penetration of topical treatment

1 Concentration
2 Viscosity: the higher the viscosity the longer the corneal contact time; ointment and gels may increase contact time and slow drug release; however, there is a lower concentration achieved in the tears compared with drops
3 Lipid solubility: the cornea is a fat–water–fat sandwich; non-ionised compounds are lipid soluble and are thus carried across the epithelium and endothelium; changing the pH may change the amount of unionised chemical but this causes more ocular discomfort and damage
4 Epithelial barrier: removal or inflammation of the epithelium improves intraocular penetration of topical medications

Factors affecting ocular penetration of systemic medications

1 Blood/ocular barriers (retina and iris): may break down in the inflamed eye
2 Protein binding: protein binding reduces amount of free drug available to tissues
3 Lipid solubility: better penetration with higher lipid solubility
4 Peak serum levels: higher peak concentrations result in greater ocular penetration
5 Low molecular weight molecules penetrate more easily; most antibiotics are large molecules

Table 17.1 The ocular autonomic system

	Sympathetic action	Parasympathetic action	Dominant receptor
Dilator pupillae	Contraction (mydriasis)	Slight relaxation	Alpha (sympathetic)
Sphincter pupillae	Slight relaxation	Contraction (miosis)	Muscarinic (parasympathetic)
Ciliary muscle	Relaxation (distance vision)	Contraction (near vision)	Muscarinic (parasympathetic)
Ciliary epithelium	Aqueous secretion	—	Beta (sympathetic)
Lacrimal gland	Slight vaso-constriction	Tear secretion	Muscarinic (parasympathetic)
Smooth muscle of the lid	Contraction	—	Alpha (sympathetic)

SYMPATHETIC SYSTEM AGONISTS

1 Adrenaline (0·5–1·0%):
  (a) actions:
      (i) α and β-receptor stimulation
      (ii) increases aqueous production
      (iii) increases rate of aqueous outflow
      (iv) mydriasis
      (v) vasoconstriction

(b) clinical uses:
- (i) open angle glaucoma
- (ii) local vasoconstriction during surgery
- (iii) delayed absorption of local anaesthetic
- (iv) keeping pupil dilated during intraocular surgery
- (v) reduction of tear secretion
- (vi) pharmacological test in Horner's syndrome

(c) side effects:
- (i) irritation
- (ii) watering
- (iii) reactive hyperaemia
- (iv) allergy
- (v) blurring of vision (mydriasis)
- (vi) black adrenochrome deposits in conjunctiva, cornea, and contact lenses
- (vii) cystoid macular oedema in aphakic patients (both intracapsular and extracapsular); reversible
- (viii) precipitation of acute angle closure glaucoma
- (ix) conjunctival fibrosis and scarring after glaucoma surgery
- (x) systemic side effects—hypertension, cardiac arrhythmias, headaches

2 Dipivefrine (0·1%):
- (a) actions:
  - (i) requires conversion by tissue enzymes to adrenaline (these enzymes are inactivated by anticholinesterases)
  - (ii) much greater corneal penetration than adrenaline ($\times 17$)
- (b) clinical uses: similar to adrenaline
- (c) side effects: similar to adrenaline but less marked because pro-drug not active until activated in tissues

3 Phenylephrine (2·5% and 10%):
- (a) actions:
  - (i) α-receptor stimulation
  - (ii) causes pupil dilatation without cycloplegia
- (b) clinical uses:
  - (i) mydriasis for fundal examination
  - (ii) ptosis in Horner's syndrome
  - (iii) senile ptosis
  - (iv) reduction of miotic induced iris cysts
  - (v) vasoconstriction of episcleral blood vessels
- (c) side effects:
  - (i) pigment release into anterior chamber
  - (ii) can cause clouding of the cornea
  - (iii) may precipitate angle closure glaucoma
  - (iv) blurring of vision (mydriasis)
  - (v) cardiovascular side effects—hypertension, bradycardia
- (d) reversed by thymoxamine

4 Cocaine (2% and 4%):
- (a) actions:
  - (i) stabilises nerve cell membranes preventing passage of ions and hence electrical conduction of "pain" impulses

    (ii) prevents re-uptake of noradrenaline by nerve terminals
  (b) clinical uses:
    (i) very effective local anaesthetic
    (ii) potentiates action of adrenaline; adrenaline also prolongs local anaesthetic action of cocaine by increasing vasoconstriction
    (iii) pharmacological test in Horner's syndrome
    (iv) paralyses parasites on eye
    (v) precipitates with iodine; has been used to cauterise dendritic ulcers
  (c) side effects:
    (i) corneal epithelial damage causing clouding of the cornea
    (ii) dilates pupil—may precipitate angle closure glaucoma; should not be used in procedures where a small pupil is required, e.g. corneal graft
5 Hydroxyamphetamine (1%):
  (a) action: causes release of noradrenaline from normal nerve terminal
  (b) clinical use: diagnostic test in Horner's syndrome
6 Apraclonidine (0·25 and 1%):
  (a) action: α_2-adrenergic agonist
  (b) clinical use: reduces intraocular pressure especially after laser trabeculoplasty and posterior capsulotomy
  (c) side effects:
    (i) dry mouth
    (ii) fatigue
    (iii) lid retraction
    (iv) mydriasis
    (v) conjunctival blanching

SYMPATHETIC SYSTEM ANTAGONISTS

1 Timolol maleate (0·25–0·5%):
  (a) actions:
    (i) non-selective β_1 and β_2-receptor blocker
    (ii) blocks cell membrane transport systems
    (iii) competes with adrenaline and noradrenaline for receptor sites
    (iv) reduces aqueous secretion
    (v) maximal action over 12 hours, but may last several weeks
  (b) clinical use: open angle glaucoma
  (c) side effects:
    (i) bronchospasm
    (ii) cardiac—arrhythmias especially bradycardia, heart failure; these may be potentiated by cardiac suppressants such as verapamil
    (iii) CNS, e.g depression
  (d) some other topical β blockers:
    (i) carteolol (1% and 2%)—partial agonist activity (intrinsic sympathomimetic activity); in theory keeps pulse rate from falling too low
    (ii) betaxolol (0·5%)—relatively cardioselective; mainly a β_1-

      receptor blocker

    (iii) levobunolol (0·25–0·5%)—non-selective β blocker

    (iv) metipranolol (0·1–0·5%)—non-selective β blocker (associated with granulomatous uveitis)

2 Thymoxamine (0·1–0·5%):

  (a) actions:

    (i) competitive α-receptor antagonist

    (ii) maximum effect in 30 min

    (iii) lasts 2 hours

  (b) clinical use: reversal of phenylephrine drops

  (c) side effects:

    (i) miosis

    (ii) transient ptosis

3 Guanethidine (5%, also 1% and 3% and with adrenaline as Ganda):

  (a) actions:

    (i) displaces noradrenaline from nerve terminals

    (ii) miosis and ptosis in 30 min

    (iii) maximum action 24 hours

  (b) clinical uses:

    (i) lid retraction in thyrotoxicosis

    (ii) open angle glaucoma in combination with adrenaline (1 + 0·2%, 3 + 0.5% as Ganda)

  (c) side effects:

    (i) miosis (initially mydriasis) ⎫

    (ii) ptosis ⎭ like a Horner's syndrome

    (iii) Ganda: 5 + 1% withdrawn as a result of cicatricial conjunctival changes

PARASYMPATHETIC AGONISTS

1 Pilocarpine (0·5–6%):

  (a) actions:

    (i) direct parasympathetic (muscarinic) agonist

    (ii) 30 min to maximum effect

    (iii) lasts 4–6 hours

    (iv) miosis

    (v) ciliary muscle contraction causing increased trabecular meshwork outflow facility and increased accommodation

    (vi) shallowing of anterior chamber

    (vii) decreased uveoscleral outflow facility

    (viii) decreased aqueous production

    (ix) increased permeability of blood–aqueous barrier

  (b) clinical uses:

    (i) glaucoma

    (ii) to reverse mydriasis (often makes vision worse)

    (iii) diagnosis of Adie's pupil (0·1%)

    (iv) for lice infestation of eyelashes

  (c) delivery forms:

    (i) drops

    (ii) with hypromellose to lessen stinging

(iii) contact lenses
(iv) membranes, e.g. Ocuserts
(v) gel
(d) side effects:
  (i) reduced visual acuity
    • miosis (particularly important effects with central lens opacities)
    • accommodation
  (ii) reduced visual fields—miosis
  (iii) allergy
  (iv) iris cysts
  (v) retinal detachment
  (vi) may precipitate pupil block glaucoma
  (vii) pupil rigidity and posterior synechiae
  (viii) brow ache
  (ix) lens opacities
  (x) punctal stenosis
  (xi) higher concentrations (4% and higher) may cause cicatrical conjunctival changes
  (xii) systemic effects:
    • sweating
    • nausea
    • vomiting
    • bradycardia
    • diarrhoea
    • salivation

2 Acetylcholine (1%):
 (a) actions:
  (i) direct stimulation of iris sphincter muscle
  (ii) rapidly broken down by anticholinesterase
  (iii) miosis lasts about 10 min
 (b) clinical uses: intraoperative miosis
 (c) side effects:
  (i) transient lens opacities caused by osmotic action
  (ii) corneal oedema
  (iii) retinal detachment
  (iv) systemic
    • bradycardia
    • hypotension

3 Methacholine (2·5%):
 (a) action: direct stimulation of parasympathetic system
 (b) clinical use: diagnosis of Adie's pupil
 (c) disadvantage: expensive

4 Carbachol (3%):
 (a) actions:
  (i) direct stimulation of parasympathetic system
  (ii) powerful miosis
  (iii) prolonged accommodative spasm
 (b) clinical use: chronic open angle glaucoma (in patients allergic to pilocarpine)

245

    (c) side effects:
        (i)   conjunctival toxicity
        (ii) similar to pilocarpine

5 Physostigmine (0·25%, 0·5%):
    (a) actions:
        (i)   reversible cholinesterase inhibitor
        (ii) miosis in 10 min, lasts 4 hours
        (iii) mild miosis may persist for several days
        (iv) ciliary spasm
    (b) clinical use: glaucoma
    (c) side effects:
        (i)   similar to pilocarpine
        (ii) eyelid twitching
        (iii) eyelid depigmentation

6 Edrophonium (10 mg/ml injection):
    (a) actions:
        (i)   reversible cholinesterase inhibitor
        (ii) improves ptosis and diplopia in myasthenia gravis for about 5 min
    (b) clinical use: diagnosis of myasthenia gravis; Tensilon test
        (i)   10 mg of edrophonium in syringe
        (ii) inject intravenous physiological saline to check placebo effect
        (iii) inject 12 mg of edrophonium and wait 1 minute
        (iv) only if no response inject rest of edrophonium
        (v) positive response is improvement in ophthalmoplegia or ptosis which relapses within minutes; intraocular pressure may also rise up to 5 mm Hg but this may only be unilateral
    (c) side effects:
        (i)   anaphylactic reaction
        (ii) cholinergic overreaction can occur in patients with myasthenia gravis after edrophonium is given; *atropine i.v. and resuscitation equipment must be readily available*

7 Ecothiopate iodide or Phospholine Iodide (0·06, 0·12, and 0·25%):
    (a) actions:
        (i)   irreversible cholinesterase inhibitor
        (ii) miosis for 24 weeks
        (iii) ciliary spasm 7 days
        (iv) fall in intraocular pressure maximal over 24 hours
    (b) clinical uses:
        (i)   chronic open angle glaucoma
        (ii) accommodative esotropia
    (c) side effects:
        (i)   *abnormal response to muscle relaxants used in general anaesthesia*
        (ii)   conjunctival vasodilatation and fibrosis
        (iii) spasm of accommodation
        (iv) corneal endothelial disturbance in high dosage
        (v)   iritis
        (vi) iris cyst formation
        (vii) cataract
        (viii) retinal detachment

(ix) eyelid twitching
(x) may precipitate pupil block glaucoma
(xi) posterior synechiae
(xii) systemic toxicity:
- CVS—bradycardia, hypertension, hypotension, and sweating
- CNS—nausea, vomiting, fatigue, paraesthesiae, insomnia, nightmares, drowsiness, muscle twitching, and coma
- gastrointestinal—salivation, abdominal cramp, and diarrhoea

PARASYMPATHETIC ANTAGONISTS

1 Atropine (1%):
  (a) actions:
    (i) competitive postganglionic muscarinic receptor blockade
    (ii) causes pupillary dilatation and cycloplegia
    (iii) decreases lacrimal secretion and vascular permeability
  (b) clinical uses:
    (i) uveitis:
- pupillary dilatation
- cycloplegia
- possible anti-inflammatory action

    (ii) cycloplegic refraction; most effective cycloplegic agent
    (iii) amblyopia (to blur vision of good eye)
    (iv) dilatation of the pupil for fundal examination where prolonged effect is required, e.g. retinal detachment
  (c) side effects:
    (i) allergy
    (ii) acute angle closure glaucoma (dilatation may also increase intraocular pressure in patients with chronic open angle glaucoma)
    (iii) blurring of vision:
- cycloplegia
- increase in optical aberrations caused by the mydriasis
- (reversal of dilatation with pilocarpine may actually worsen vision in some patients)

    (iv) systemic reactions:
- tachycardia
- facial flush
- tremor
- dryness of mouth and skin
- delirium

(these occur particularly in elderly and young patients; for a 4·5 kg child a lethal dose is 10 mg (20 drops of a 1% solution))

2 Hyoscine (0·25 and 0·5%): similar to atropine but shorter acting
3 Homatropine (1–2%): similar to atropine but shorter acting

4 Lachesine (1%): maximum mydriatic action at 1 hour and lasts 5–6 hours; useful if patient allergic to atropine
5 Cyclopentolate (0·5–2%): shorter acting than homatropine but better cycloplegic; useful for short term dilatation of pupil and cycloplegia
6 Tropicamide (0·5–1%): short acting with only partial cycloplegia; useful for short term dilatation of the pupil
7 Combination of drugs for dilatation of the pupil: Mydricaine No. 2 = atropine 1 mg, adrenaline 0·12 ml, 1:1000 solution, and procaine 6·0 mg, made up to 0·3 ml volume; given subconjunctivally to dilate the pupil; relatively large dose of atropine so caution in:
   (a) elderly people
   (b) young patients
   (c) patients who may need bilateral injections
       (smaller dose ampoule available (Mydricaine No. 1) which has half the concentration of Mydricaine No. 2)]

Table 17.2

Drug	Mydriasis		Cycloplegia	
	Max effect (min)	Recovery (days)	Max effect (hours)	Recovery (days)
Atropine	45	10	6	14
Hyoscine	35	7	1	7
Homatropine	60	3	1	3
Cyclopentolate	60	1	1	1
Tropicamide	40	0·25	0·5	0·25

CARBONIC ANHYDRASE INHIBITORS

1 Acetazolamide (oral):
   (a) actions:
       (i) inhibition of carbonic anhydrase activity
       (ii) reduces the bicarbonate in the aqueous humour and the water secreted with it
       (iii) fall in intraocular pressure of 30–60%
       (iv) action over 6–12 hours after oral treatment; duration of action can be prolonged by sustained release capsules
   (b) clinical uses:
       (i) reduction of intraocular pressure
       (ii) reduction of intracranial pressure
       (iii) "mountain sickness" (prophylaxis)
       (iv) macular oedema
   (c) side effects:
       (i) malaise
       (ii) anorexia
       (iii) nausea
       (iv) depression

(v) paraesthesiae
(vi) transient myopia
(vii) hypokalaemia
(viii) metabolic acidosis
(ix) renal stones
(x) deafness in patients with Ménière's disease
(xi) allergic reaction including Stevens–Johnson syndrome
2 Dorzolamide (topical):
  (a) actions:
    (i) similar to acetazolamide
    (ii) penetrates sclera and cornea getting to ciliary body (reaches ciliary body before aqueous)
  (b) clinical uses:
    (i) reduction of intraocular pressure
  (c) side effects:
    (i) local—include stinging, burning, foreign body sensation, bitter taste in mouth, tearing (common because of low pH), and allergies; no effect of pupil size or accommodation
    (ii) systemic—theoretically same as acetazolamide, although only one case of renal stones reported to date

TOPICAL NON-STEROIDAL ANTI-INFLAMMATORY AGENTS

1 Flurbiprofen sodium:
  (a) actions:
    (i) competes with arachidonic acid for cyclo-oxygenase binding
    (ii) prevents arachidonic acid converting to prostaglandin
    (iii) may prevent vasodilatation, breakdown of the blood–aqueous humour barrier, intraoperative miosis, and increased intra-ocular pressure
  (b) clinical uses:
    (i) prevention of miosis during intraocular surgery
    (ii) reduction of ocular inflammation, e.g. episcleritis, post-operative
    (iii) prevention of cystoid macular oedema (after cataract surgery)
2 Mast cell stabilisers, e.g. sodium cromoglycate (drops 2%, ointment 4%), nedocromil sodium (drops 2%):
  (a) actions:
    (i) inhibition of mast cell degranulation, the local release of vasoactive amines, and inflammatory agents
    (ii) stabilises mast cell membrane and modulates the intracellular events that lead to mast cell degranulation
  (b) clinical uses:
    (i) hayfever conjunctivitis
    (ii) recurrent allergic conjunctivitis
    (iii) perennial allergic conjunctivitis
    (iv) vernal keratoconjunctivitis
    (v) giant papillary conjunctivitis
    (vi) ligneous conjunctivitis

TOPICAL PROSTAGLANDIN ANALOGUES

Latanoprost (0·006%) phenyl substituted prostaglandin $F_{2\alpha}$ analogue

1 Actions: increases uveoscleral outflow of aqueous
2 Clinical uses: reduction of intraocular pressure
3 Side effects:
   (a) local effects, including irritation and foreign body sensation
   (b) increased iris pigmentation

PUPIL TESTS IN HORNER'S SYNDROME

1 Adrenaline 0·1% test:
   (a) relies on denervation hypersensitivity
   (b) not present immediately after sympathetic chain damage occurs
2 Cocaine 4% test:
   (a) prevents re-uptake of noradrenaline by nerve terminals of the dilator pupillae muscle
   (b) observe 30 min after instillation
   (c) test is dose dependent; if there is epithelial damage (e.g. from applanation), this may enhance cocaine entry and cause spurious dilatation
3 Hydroxyamphetamine 1% test:
   (a) causes release of noradrenaline from the normal nerve terminal
   (b) observe 30 min after instillation, but may take up to 2 hours to work in patients with heavily pigmented irides
   (c) should not be done within 2 days of cocaine test as cocaine blocks the uptake of hydroxyamphetamine at nerve terminals

Table 17.3 Pharmacological pupil tests

		Condition		
	Normal	Central Horner's syndrome	Postganglionic Horner's syndrome	Primary iris disease
Drops:				
Adrenaline 0·1%	No change	No change	Full dilatation	No change
Cocaine 4%	Full dilatation	Partial dilatation	No change	No change
Hydroxyamphetamine 1%	Full dilatation	Full dilatation	No change	No change

OTHER PUPIL DIAGNOSTIC TESTS

1 Drug induced pupillary dilatation:
   (a) theory:
      (i) drugs that paralyse the sphincter do so by blocking the muscarinic receptor sites
      (ii) a weak pilocarpine solution cannot bind with enough receptors to cause pupillary constriction
   (b) technique:

(i) apply 0·5% pilocarpine to each eye

(ii) observe after 30 min

(c) positive result: failure of the pupil to constrict; this suggests drug induced pupillary dilatation; a traumatic mydriasis will also be unresponsive

2 Adie's myotonic pupil:

(a) theory:

(i) denervation hypersensitivity occurs after damage to the para-sympathetic nerve supply to the pupil

(ii) denervation hypersensitivity is not immediately present

(b) technique:

(i) 0·1% pilocarpine to each eye

(ii) observe after 20 min

(iii) (methacholine 2·5% may also be used but this is expensive and has to be freshly prepared)

(c) positive result: constriction of a previously dilated pupil

SOME OCULAR SIDE EFFECTS OF SYSTEMIC DRUGS

1 Eyelids/cornea/conjunctiva:

(a) phenothiazines, e.g. chlorpromazine; discoloration of the skin and golden-brown granules in the conjunctiva and fine deposits in the cornea

(b) Stevens–Johnson syndrome secondary to hypersensitivity from drugs such as sulphonamides

(c) oculomucocutaneous syndrome secondary to practolol

(d) chloroquine: deposition in the corneal epithelium sometimes in a whorl like appearance (verticillata); causes hazy vision, photo-phobia, and haloes around lights

(e) amiodarone: skin photosensitivity and corneal verticillata

(f) gold: fine particles in the conjunctiva or cornea

2 Lens:

(a) corticosteroids: posterior subcapsular lens opacities (and open angle glaucoma)

(b) phenothiazines, e.g. chlorpromazine: fine yellowish-brown granules beneath the anterior lens capsule

(c) myopia from tetracyclines, sulphonamides, acetazolamide, and antihistamines

3 Pupil:

(a) pupillary dilatation may precipitate angle closure glaucoma after treatment with atropine, anti-parkinsonian agents, and cyclotropic drugs

(b) miosis: particularly with opiates

4 Retina:

(a) chloroquine compounds: these have an affinity for melanin; early visual complaints include blurring of vision, photophobia, and flashes of light; bilateral retinal changes start with an abnormal foveal reflex and parafoveal pigmentary disturbance; this leads to a "bull's eye" appearance

(b) phenothiazines, e.g. thioridazine: acute onset with diminution of vision, retinal oedema, and hyperaemia of the optic disc; chronic onset with a fine pigment scatter in the central area of the fundus extending peripherally; the pigment coalesces into plaques

(c) oxygen: high oxygen concentrations are implicated in the retinopathy of prematurity

(d) tamoxifen: retinal pigmentation, especially parafoveal; tamoxifen deposition

(e) canthaxanthin (Orobronze) oral tanning agent: refractive deposits in retina

5 Optic nerve:
  (a) anti-tuberculosis drugs:
    (i) streptomycin—xanthopsia with central scotoma
    (ii) ethambutol:
      • visual loss with colour vision defects especially to green
      • optic neuritis
      • greater risk of ocular toxicity with renal dysfunction
      • pyridoxine may help to protect from toxicity
  (b) chloramphenicol: occurs most frequently in children; disc hyperaemia with haemorrhages and oedema
  (c) tetracycline: benign intracranial hypertension and papilloedema
  (d) digitalis: disturbance of colour vision, usually sensation of yellow coloration (xanthopsia)
  (e) penicillamine: optic neuritis
  (f) quinine is probably directly toxic with secondary vascular closure
  (g) clioquinol (Entero-Vioform): optic neuritis especially in Japanese
6 Ocular motility:
  (a) carbamazepine and phenytoin: nystagmus
  (b) streptomycin: paralysis of eye muscles and nystagmus
  (c) phenothiazines and metoclopramide: oculogyric crisis

18
OPTICS

LIGHT

1 Visible spectrum: 400 nm (blue) to 780 nm (red)
2 Theories of light:
   (a) particle theory (Planck): quanta of energy proportional to wavelength
   (b) wave theory (Maxwell):
      (i) energy passage through medium
      (ii) particle vibration perpendicular to direction of wave
      (iii) amplitude (maximal displacement)
      (iv) wavelength: distance between symmetrical points

Interference

1 Constructive: summation when waves in phase
2 Destructive: algebraic summation when waves out of phase, e.g. in corneal stroma, anti-reflective coatings

Diffraction

1 Production of secondary wavefronts after passage of light through slits or around edges
2 Resulting interference (Airy's discs) limits resolution through aperture

Polarisation

1 All waves in same plane
2 Polarising substances transmit in only one plane
3 Polarising angle = incident angle producing polarised reflection
4 Uses of polarising filters:
   (a) reduction of glare, e.g. sunglasses
   (b) assessment of binocular vision, e.g. Titmus fly
   (c) checking of stress lines in lens manufacture

Photometry

1 Quantitative measurement of light
2 Luminous flux: total emission (lumens)

3 Luminous intensity: emission in given direction (candela)
4 Illumination: inverse square law:

$$E = \frac{I \times \cos\ i}{d^2}$$

I = luminous intensity (candela)
d = distance from source
i = angle of incidence
5 Luminance: measurement of reflected light

Laws of reflection

1 Incident ray, reflected ray, and normal in same plane
2 Angle of reflection equals angle of incidence

Reflection at a plane mirror

1 Image virtual
2 Image laterally transposed
3 Image distance equals object distance
4 Magnification equals unity

Reflection at a spherical surface

1 Centre of curvature (C)
2 Centre of mirror = principal point (P)
3 CP = principal axis
4 $\frac{1}{2}$ CP = principal focus (F)
5 Object distance = u
6 Image distance = v
7 Focal distance = f
8 Rays parallel to CP are reflected through F
9 Rays incident to C are reflected back along path

mirror formula: $\dfrac{1}{f} = \dfrac{1}{v} - \dfrac{1}{u}$

magnification (M) = image size/object size = v/u

10 Uses:
   (a) catoptric imagery (Purkinje images 1–4)
   (b) keratometers
   (c) Placido's disc

Refraction

1 Change in direction of wavefront on traversing media of different optical densities (n_1, n_2)
2 Velocity of light varies with optical density
3 Refractive index (n) is the ratio of velocities in air and medium
4 Snell's laws:
   (a) incident angle (i), refracted angle (r), and normal are in the same

plane

(b) refractive index $(n) = \sin i / \sin r$

5 Refraction through a plate of glass: emergent ray is parallel to incident ray

6 Critical angle: ray emerging from optically dense medium refracted away from normal; at critical angle ray refracted along interface; at greater angles total internal reflection occurs

7 Dispersion: refractive index of medium varies with wavelength; results in separation of wavelengths

8 Dispersive power of a medium is not related to refractive index

9 Refraction at a curved surface produces vergence:

surface (vergence) power $= (n_2 - n_1)/\text{radius}$

PRISMS

1 Portion of refracting surface bordered by 2 planes inclined at an angle α (refracting angle or apical angle)

2 Axis = bisection of refracting angle

3 Base = opposite side to refracting angle

4 Deviation (D) proportional to:
   (a) refractive index
   (b) refracting angle
   (c) angle of incidence

5 Prisms calibrated in position of minimum deviation: angle of incidence equals angle of refraction

6 Ophthalmic prisms are right angle prisms calibrated with angled incidence at 90° = Prentice position

7 Glass prisms: $D = \alpha/2$

8 Prism power measured in prism dioptres (Δ); 1 dioptre (D) = 1 cm linear deviation at 1 m

9 Image:
   (a) erect
   (b) virtual
   (c) displaced to apex

Uses of prisms

1 Diagnostic:
   (a) measurement of angle of strabismus objectively by prism cover test
   (b) measurement of strabismus subjectively by Maddox rod
   (c) assessment of possible diplopia after proposed strabismus surgery
   (d) measurement of fusional reserve
   (e) assessment of microtropia (4 Δ test)
   (f) assessment of simulated blindness

2 Instruments:
   (a) slitlamp/operating microscope (Porro prism inverts inverted image)
   (b) keratometer (Wollaston prism)
   (c) pachymeter
   (d) applanation tonometer

3 Therapeutic:

(a) convergence insufficiency
(b) relieve diplopia

Special prisms

1 Fresnel prism: 2 mm thick strip of plastic; multiple prisms produce effect of single large prism with equivalent refracting angle
2 Reflecting prisms:
   (a) Porro: deviates light 180° and inverts image
   (b) dove: inverts image
3 Wollaston prism: two quartz prisms (a double refractor) placed at 90°, producing two beams at a fixed angle

LENSES

1 Portion of a refracting medium bordered by 2 curved surfaces with a common axis
2 Total vergence depends on the power of each surface vergence and lens thickness
3 Sign convention:

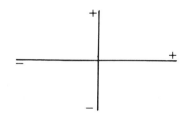

Thin lens theory

1 Ignores lens thickness
2 Optical centre of lens = nodal point (N)
3 Centres of curvature of surfaces = C_1, C_2
4 Principal axis (p) = $C_1 \, N \, C_2$
5 Principal foci lie on p = F_1, F_2
6 Principal plane (P) perpendicular to principal axis at nodal point
7 Focal length = principal plane to F_2 (f)
8 Power of lens (D) = algebraic sum of vergence power; reciprocal of P; positive for convex lenses; negative for concave lenses
9 Magnification:

   linear = image size/object size = v/u

   angular = angle subtended by image/angle subtended by object

10 Magnification with simple loupe: assuming working distance of 25 cm: $M = F/4$, where F = lens power (D)

11 Thin lens formula: $\dfrac{1}{f_2} = \dfrac{1}{v} - \dfrac{1}{u}$

12 Prismatic effect of decentration: peripheral portions of a lens act as prisms with increasing refracting angle: $P = F \times d$, where $P = \Delta$, $F =$ lens power, $d =$ decentration in cm; uses:
   (a) instead of actual prism addition
   (b) up to 5 mm of displacement
   (c) decentration along axis of astigmatic lenses has no prismatic effect

Astigmatic lenses

1 Cylindrical lens:
   (a) vergence power in one meridian only
   (b) axis of cylinder perpendicular to power meridian
   (c) production of line image of point source, parallel to axis
2 Toric lens:
   (a) cylindrical lens superimposed on spherical lens; produces blurred image within Sturm's conoid
   (b) circle of least confusion = point of maximum definition

Identification of lenses

1 Viewing through lens:
   (a) direction of apparent movement of object on moving lens:
       (i) against = convex lens
       (ii) with = concave lens
   (b) apparent displacement on rotating lens = astigmatic lens:
       (i) find position of no displacement
       (ii) check direction of apparent movement in each meridian
       (iii) mark lens on each axis to locate optical centre
       (iv) constant displacement = prismatic incorporation
2 Neutralisation: using opposite lens power to neutralise apparent movements
3 Lens measure (e.g. Geneva): refractive index required to calculate power
4 Focimeter:
   (a) measures vertex power
   (b) measures astigmatic powers and axes
   (c) allows optical centre marking and prism assessment

Lens shape

1 Round (disadvantage of requiring lens lock to prevent rotation)
2 Round oval
3 Long oval
4 Pantoscopic (oval with flattened top)

Lens section

1 Symmetrical: simple lenses
2 Asymmetrical:
   (a) best form lenses: usually meniscus shaped to reduce aberrations:

     (i) −6 D posterior curve, up to +7 D lens power
    (ii) +6 D anterior curve, up to −6 D lens power
   (iii) +1·25 D anterior curve, −6 to −10 D lens power
   (iv) plano anterior curve, −10 to −20 D lens power
(b) periscopic lenses: 1·25 D base curve
(c) aspheric lenses: flatter peripherally to reduce power and aberrations
(d) lenticular: lens power located centrally; reduces weight and aberrations
(e) variable focus lenses: changing lens section to increase power in downgaze

Bifocal lenses

1 Forms:
  (a) Franklin split = two piece
  (b) cemented ⎫
  (c) fused   ⎬ segments
  (d) solid   ⎭
2 Shape:
  (a) 22 or 24 mm round segments
  (b) 38 or 45 mm round segments
  (c) 25 or 28 mm straight top segments (D segment)
  (d) executive segments
3 Relative indications:
  (a) high AC/A ratio esotropia
  (b) convenience
4 Relative contraindications:
  (a) anisometropia
  (b) high oblique astigmatism
  (c) heterophoria
  (d) reading add more than 4 D
5 Intolerance:
  (a) related to segment size, height, power
  (b) chromatic aberration (fused segments)
  (c) prismatic jump:
    (i) if insert not concentric
    (ii) reduced with executive and D segments
  (d) sudden changes in focal power
  (e) oblique astigmatism: near visual axis and near segment optical axis not coincident
  (f) muscle imbalance: caused by reduced accommodative convergence
  (g) lack of intermediate focus

Trifocal lenses

1 Intermediate power:
  (a) usually $\frac{1}{2}$ power reading segment
  (b) 8 mm in depth
2 Shape:
  (a) D segment

(b) executive segment
3 Varifocal lenses:
  (a) progressive power increase from top to bottom
  (b) small corridor of intermediate power
  (c) peripheral distortion
  (d) intolerance especially in high astigmatism or high reading addition

Lens aberrations (distortions in the image produced)

1 Chromatic:
  (a) related to dispersion of light
  (b) reduced by combining lens of high refractive index/low dispersive power with lens of low refractive index/high dispersive power to produce required refraction
2 Spherical: prismatic effect of peripheral lens resulting in increasing deviation:
  (a) reduced by:
      (i) best form lenses
      (ii) diaphragm to exclude peripheral lens
      (iii) lenticular lenses
      (iv) aspheric lenses
      (v) doublets
  (b) reduced in eye by:
      (i) peripheral corneal flattening
      (ii) iris stop
      (iii) lower refractive index of lens cortex compared with nucleus
      (iv) Stiles–Crawford effect
3 Oblique: oblique light, not parallel to principal axis; causes astigmatic refraction:
  (a) reduced by:
      (i) keeping incident light parallel to axis
      (ii) diaphragm to exclude peripheral lens
      (iii) best form lenses
  (b) reduced in eye by:
      (i) aplanatic cornea
      (ii) curved retina
      (iii) poor resolution of peripheral cornea
      (iv) iris stop
4 Coma: unequal magnification of object resulting from object not being on principal axis
5 Image distortion:
  (a) barrel from concave lens
  (b) pincushion from convex lens
6 Curvature of field: plane object produces curved image

Thick lens theory

1 Lens thickness must be taken into account
2 Principles to simplify formulae:
  (a) 2 principal planes (P_1, P_2; perpendicular to principal axis; light parallel to axis incident on first plane is projected to focal point as if leaving from second plane

(b) 2 nodal points (N_1, N_2; points on principal axis; light incident on N_1 leaves system as if from N_2 and parallel to the incident ray
3 True focal lengths:
  (a) $P_1 F_1 = f_1$
  (b) $P_2 F_2 = f_2$
4 Vertex focal length: measure from lens surface to focal point
5 Back vertex power: reciprocal of vertex focal length; different from equivalent or true power

Reduced eye (after Listing)

1 Single principal plane and nodal point
2 Distances from anterior cornea:
  (a) principal plane $+1\cdot35$ mm
  (b) nodal point $+7\cdot08$ mm
  (c) F_1: $-15\cdot70$ mm
  (d) F_2: $+24\cdot13$ mm
  (e) lens power: $+15$ D
  (f) aphakic power: $+43$ D
  (g) F_1 aphakic eye: $-21\cdot88$ mm

OPTICS OF EMMETROPIA AND AMETROPIA

1 Emmetropia: axial length equals dioptric power of eye with far point at infinity
2 States of emmetropia: as a result of appropriate matching of axial length and refractive power far point can remain at infinity
3 Myopia: finite far point
4 Hypermetropia: virtual far point
5 Types of ametropia:
  (a) axial
  (b) curvature
  (c) index

Accommodation

1 Ability of the eye to change its refractive power to maintain focus on an approaching object
2 Near point: point of nearest distinct vision
3 Range: far point to near point
4 Amplitude: change in dioptric power
5 Reducing amplitude with age:
  (a) 14 D as infant
  (b) 4 D at 45 years
  (c) 1 D at 60 years
6 Presbyopia discomfort/difficulty for near vision due to age related reduction in amplitude of accommodation

Ocular astigmatism

1 Variation of refraction in different meridians
2 Regular: axes perpendicular:

(a) with the rule: negative cylinder horizontal

(b) against the rule: negative cylinder vertical

(c) oblique: regular—axes at 90° to each other

3 Classification:
  (a) simple: one axis emmetropic
  (b) compound: both axes ametropic
  (c) mixed: each axis of opposite power
4 Bioblique: axes not at right angles
5 Irregular
  (a) no axes determinable
  (b) corneal or lenticular pathology

Optical correction of ametropia

1 Using lenses such that rays appear to come from the far point of the eye
2 If lens positioned close to the eye then far point equals focal length of the lens

Effective power

1 If lens position is altered, far point and focal point no longer coincide; effective power of lens thus changes
2 On moving lens away from eye:
  (a) positive lenses: power effectively increases
  (b) negative lenses: power effectively decreases
3 Effect of position significant if lens power is greater than 5 D
4 Back vertex distance = distance between the back of the lens and the corneal apex
5 Power of new lens (F_2): $F_2 = F_1/(1 - dF_1)$, where d = distance of change in metres

Relative spectacle magnification (RSM)

1 RSM = corrected image size/emmetropic image size
2 Axial ametropia: RSM = 1 if correcting lens at anterior focal point
3 Index ametropia:
  (a) RSM = 1 if lens at principal plane of eye.

(b) hypermetropia, RSM > 1 (with spectacles).

(c) myopia, RSM < 1 (with spectacles); RSM tends to unity on approaching eye

4 RSM and aphakia:

(a) spectacles, RSM = 1·36

(b) contact lens, RSM = 1·1

(c) intraocular lens, RSM = 1·0

Anisometropia

1 Difference in refractive state between the two eyes

2 Causes:

(a) congenital

(b) acquired, e.g. nuclear sclerosis, lens dislocation, and extraction

3 Hypermetropia > 1 D associated with amblyopia

4 Anisometropia > 2·50 D produces a 5% image disparity

Aniseikonia

1 Different image size in each eye

2 Measured with Goldmann eikonometer

3 No binocular single vision possible if there is more than a 5% disparity of image

4 Iseikonic lenses:

(a) change image size

(b) ability relates to lens thickness and anterior curve

(c) 5% maximum change in image size

(d) thick, heavy

(e) difficult to manufacture

(f) expensive

Optical problems with spectacle correction of aphakia

1 Increased image size:

(a) sensation of proximity and misjudgment of distance

(b) patients feel small

(c) image distortion (pincushion effect)

2 Aniseikonia with unilateral aphakia

3 Prismatic effects:

(a) ring scotoma

(b) "Jack in the box" phenomenon

4 Narrow field of vision

5 Spectacle weight and cost

6 Cosmetic

INDICATIONS FOR CONTACT LENSES

1 Optical (NHS eligibility):

(a) there must be definite improvement over spectacle corrected vision; final decision by consultant

(b) ametropia of 10·00 D or more

(c) aniseikonia of 10% or more

(d) anisometropia of 4·00 D or more
(e) corneal irregularities: keratoconus, corneal scarring, and astigmatism
(f) therapeutic soft lenses
(g) part of telescopic lens system
(h) ocular pathology:
    (i) albinism
    (ii) aniridia
    (iii) coloboma
    (iv) ptosis
2 Diagnostic:
  (a) contact lenses for examination and treatment, e.g. 3 mirror, gonio, and panfundus lenses
  (b) radio-opaque localising lens
  (c) electrodiagnostic lenses
  (d) lens for specular microscopy
3 Occupational:
  (a) sports
  (b) acting
4 Cosmetic:
  (a) heterochromia
  (b) phthisis
5 Protective: shield in radiotherapy
6 Therapeutic:
  (a) bandage lens: a soft high water content lens:
    (i) bullous keratopathy
    (ii) trichiasis
    (iii) trauma
    (iv) descemetocele
    (v) prevention of erosions
    (vi) ulcer healing
    (vii) small leaking wound
    (viii) filamentary keratitis
  (b) haptic lens:
    (i) prevention of symblepharon
    (ii) ptosis, e.g. in progressive external ophthalmoplegia
  (c) soft lens soaked in drug for prolonged delivery, e.g. methazolamide

Types of loupes

1 Hand held
2 Stand magnifier
3 Paper weight
4 Lens bars

Some non-optical devices for poor vision

1 Large print books
2 Good lighting
3 Large fibre tip pens

4 Large dial telephones
5 Large playing cards, etc
6 Projection systems including closed circuit TV

Galilean telescope

1 Convex objective, concave eye piece
2 Separated by difference in focal length
3 Magnification = power of eyepiece (F_e)/power of objective (F_o)
4 Compact system
5 Erect image
6 Minimal distortion
7 May be adapted for near or distance
8 Can be spectacle mounted
9 Field of view:
   (a) depends on size of objective
   (b) has an inverse relationship to magnification
   (c) increases with proximity to the eye
   (d) increases as distance between lenses is reduced

Compound microscope

1 Convex objective and eyepiece
2 Separated by distance greater than focal combined lengths
3 Image inverted

Direct ophthalmoscope

1 Field of view:
   (a) about 6°
   (b) related to:
      (i) size of sight hole:
         • mirror
         • observer's pupil
         • subject's pupil
      (ii) state of ametropia:
         • myopia (small field)
         • hypermetropia (large field)
   (c) increases with proximity of ophthalmoscope to subject
2 Retinal image size:
   (a) image larger in myopia
   (b) image smaller in hypermetropia
3 Magnification (simple loupe): $M = 60/4 = \times 15$

Indirect ophthalmoscope

1 Field of illumination:
   (a) related to state of ametropia:
      (i) myopia, large field
      (ii) hypermetropia, smaller field
   (b) related to subject's pupil size

2 Field of view:
   (a) about 25° field
   (b) related to:
      (i) aperture of condensing lens
      (ii) size of observer's pupil
3 Retinal image:
   (a) magnification:
      (i) using $+13\,D = \times 5$
      (ii) using $+20\,D = \times 3$
   (b) change in image size on moving lens is related to ametropic state; on moving away:
      (i) emmetropia—remains the same
      (ii) myopia—increases
      (iii) hypermetropia—decreases
   (c) using binocular ophthalmoscope stereoscopic view obtained
   (d) ametropia has relatively little effect on image size
   (e) image inverted vertically and horizontally

Measurement of corneal curvature

1 Placido's disc
2 Keratometer: measures central zone; 2 types:
   (a) Von Helmholtz: fixed object size (O); image size (I) measured (rotating glass plates)
   (b) Javal–Schiötz: fixed image size (I); object size (O) varied (mires on curved side arms)
   (c) corneal radius $(r) = 2uI/O$, where u = focal distance of viewing telescope (constant)

Slitlamp

1 Binocular microscope coupled to projection system
2 Results in:
   (a) common axis of rotation
   (b) microscope and projector having coincident foci
   (c) axis of rotation at this common point
   (d) long working distance which allows access

Slitlamp examination techniques
1 Direct focal illumination
2 Diffuse illumination
3 Retroillumination
4 Lateral illumination
5 Specular reflection
6 Sclerotic scatter
7 Blue or green filter
8 Additional techniques for fundal examination:
   (a) Hruby lens: $-58 \cdot 6D$
   (b) contact lenses: plano concave
   (c) indirect lenses: $+90, +78D$

Applanation tonometer

1 Produces image splitting to ensure standardised fluorescein ring size
2 Produced by prisms with bases in opposite directions

Pachymeter

1 For the measurement of:
 (a) corneal thickness
 (b) anterior chamber depth
2 Uses Purkinje–Sanson image:
 (a) image I (anterior corneal surface)
 (b) image II (posterior corneal surface)
 (c) image III (anterior lens surface)
  (images I and II to measure corneal thickness; images II and III to measure anterior chamber depth)
3 Types:
 (a) Maurice and Giardine: splits incident light
 (b) Jaeger: special eyepiece

REFRACTION PROCEDURE

1 Measurement of monocular vision with and without correction
2 Cover test with and without correction
3 Measurement of interpupillary distance (IPD)
4 Place trial frame on patient and adjust IPD
5 Direct patient's gaze at distant target and carry out retinoscopy:
 (a) in presence of strabismus occlude fellow eye
 (b) in young fog fellow eye with plus lens: fog patients with latent nystagmus rather than occlude
6 Subtract the reciprocal of the working distance in metres from the result
7 Subjective procedure in each eye:
 (a) monocular vision with corrected retinoscopy result (working distance subtracted)
 (b) check best vision sphere with Snellen chart or duochrome
 (c) correct astigmatism with either Jackson's cross cylinder or fan and block; check axis before power of cylinder
 (d) recheck best vision sphere (aiming for maximum plus or minimum minus)
 (e) repeat procedure for fellow eye
8 Binocular balance (to equalise accommodative state): Humphrey, Septum, 1 dioptre blur back
9 Oculomotor and accommodation tests:
 (a) distance heterophoria by Maddox rod
 (b) measure amplitude of accommodation, monocular, and binocular; calculate near addition; adjust trial frame IPD
 (c) measure near heterophoria by Maddox wing
 (d) measure near point of convergence
 (e) additional tests may be used if appropriate:
  (i) cover test

(ii) fixation disparity
(iii) AC/A ratio
(iv) fusional reserves
 (v) stereopsis
(vi) colour tests

RETINOSCOPY

1 Small proportion of light entering eye is reflected; this is brought to a focus at the far point of the eye
2 Observation of the movement of this image produced by movement of the light source allows location of this far point
3 Three stages:
(a) illumination: using a light source reflected via a plane or concave mirror
(b) reflex: image formation at far point
(c) projection: location of the far point
4 Point of reversal: end point of retinoscopy after inserting trial lenses; far point is located at nodal point of examiner's eye
5 Observed movements using plane mirror:
(a) against: myopia of greater than working distance
(b) with:
(i) emmetropia.
(ii) myopia of less than working distance.
(iii) hypermetropia
6 Very accurate technique
7 Errors relate to age:
(a) young, $+0.5$ D as a result of reflection at inner limiting membrane
(b) old, -0.5 D caused by reflection from deeper layers
8 Correction of astigmatism: check movement in principal meridians and correct with trial lenses using spheres or spherocylinder form

Subjective techniques

1 Pin hole test:
(a) reduces the size of the blur circle improving resolution
(b) allows rapid differentiation between reduced vision caused by ametropia and that caused by pathology or amblyopia
(c) vision not fully corrected if ametropia greater than ± 4.00 D
2 Best vision sphere (BVS): best spherical correcting lens to provide best visual acuity; minimum minus, maximum plus technique
3 Duochrome test:
(a) assessment of BVS
(b) uses ocular chromatic aberrations; shorter wavelength green light refracted more than red
(c) red and green targets used
(d) should be used with other methods of BVS testing
(e) first impression of target clarity important:
(i) emmetropic individual—equally bright targets
(ii) myopic individual—red more distinct

(iii) hypermetropic individual—usually green more distinct; may accommodate to either

(f)   can be used if the patient is colour blind

Jackson's cross cylinder

1 Spherocylindrical lens in which the power of the sphere is half the power of the cylinder and of the opposite sign
2 Powers: + 0·25 to + 2·00 D
3 Uses:
   (a) axis determination
   (b) determination of cylinder power
   (c) to confirm absence of cylinder
4 Only of use if close to real cylinder on retinoscopy
5 Encourage active accommodation and use circular targets one line above vision line on acuity chart
6 Check axis, then power and then axis again
7 Change of 0·5 D in cylinder requires the addition of a 0·25 D sphere of the opposite sign

Stenopaic slit

1 Restricts blur circle in one meridian
2 Subjective technique for correction of astigmatism using BVS technique

Fan and block

Technique for determining the power and axis of cylinder.

APPENDIX I

PHOTOCOAGULATION

Relies on the absorption of light energy by ocular pigments such as xanthophyll (maximum at lower wavelengths), melanin, and haemoglobin (maximum at lower wavelengths). Light energy is converted into heat. Source of light can be:

1 Bright light, e.g. xenon arc lamp
2 Laser = light amplification by stimulated emission of radiation

Indications for photocoagulation

1 Anterior segment:
   (a) eyelid tumours: removed with the carbon dioxide laser
   (b) destroying eyelash roots in trichiasis
   (c) cutting sutures
   (d) trabeculoplasty in primary open angle glaucoma
   (e) iridotomy
   (f) pupilloplasty
   (g) photocoagulation of the ciliary processes to reduce aqueous secretion
   (h) photocoagulation of blood vessels on cornea and iris
   (i) gonioplasty
2 Posterior segment:
   (a) creating adhesions around retinal holes and tears and prophylaxis of retinal degenerations, e.g. lattice
   (b) panretinal photocoagulation for proliferative retinal disease and rubeosis iridis
   (c) macular oedema: focal grid laser in diabetes, retinal vein occlusion
   (d) central serous maculopathy (improves speed of resolution but not visual prognosis)
   (e) direct photocoagulation to vascular abnormalities: including vascular malformations (von Hippel–Lindau syndrome), choroidal neovascular membranes, persistent extrachoroidal neovascular complexes
   (f) intraocular tumours

Complications of photocoagulation

To patient

1 Cornea:
   (a) burns
   (b) erosions
   (c) superficial punctate keratopathy or keratitis: neurotrophic keratopathy with trans-scleral diode laser cycloablation
   (d) bullous keratopathy:
2 Iris:
   (a) burns to iris causing iritis
   (b) iris atrophy
   (c) sphincter damage
3 Lens: lens opacities
4 Anterior chamber: shallowing of anterior chamber as a result of ciliochoroidal detachment, which may lead to closed angle glaucoma
5 Posterior segment:
   (a) foveal burn
   (b) retinal and choroidal haemorrhage
   (c) macular oedema and pucker
   (d) occlusion of vein or artery
   (e) contraction of fibrous tissue
   (f) night blindness
   (g) change in colour perception
   (h) constriction of visual fields
   (i) nerve fibre bundle defects
   (j) decrease in visual acuity
   (k) subretinal neovascularisation
   (l) enlargement of scar over time with loss of central acuity

To operator

1 Inadvertent exposure: retinal burns
2 Tritan colour deficiency with prolonged/repeated use of argon blue–green

Argon laser

1 Principle: blue–green light 488 nm and green light 515 nm; absorbed by melanin, haemoglobin, and xanthophyll; green wavelength may be advantageous in the macular area as a result of reduced absorption by xanthophyll. Less operator injury with green wavelength
2 Clinical uses: as above; most frequently used ophthalmic laser, but diode beginning to supersede in several areas

Krypton laser

1 Principle: red light, 647 nm; absorbed by melanin, poorly by haemoglobin and xanthophyll; theoretical advantage over argon:
   (a) less absorbed by xanthophyll in mature lens and macula
   (b) less absorbed by vitreous haemorrhage
2 Clinical uses: predominantly retinal and macular photocoagulation

(however, little evidence that wavelength critical in retinal photo-coagulation)

Carbon dioxide laser

1 Principle: high absorptive properties
2 Clinical uses:
   (a) lid tumours
   (b) trabeculosclerostomy (hole in sclera and trabecular meshwork)
   (c) vaporising intraocular tumours
   (d) closed end CO_2 laser probe for cauterising bleeding blood vessels or creating choroidoretinal adhesions around a tear

Neodymium:yttrium–aluminium–garnet (Nd:YAG) laser

1 Principle: 1064 nm, infrared non-visible light; main use in ophthalmology is high power pulses causing optical breakdown and localised mechanical disruptions; this process does not rely on light absorption so semi-transparent membranes can be cut; high power pulses can be one of two modalities:
   (a) q (quality) switched: usual pulse duration 10–20 ns, energy up to 20 mJ; several pulses can be used in a single burst
   (b) mode locked: train of pulses delivered lasting picoseconds (typically 30 ps); each train has 7–10 pulses with interspace pulsing of 5–7 ns; whole train lasts 35–70 ns; mode locking is now rarely used
   (c) the Nd:YAG laser can also be used at longer exposure duration and low peak power (free running); no optical breakdown and purely thermal interactions; exposure durations 0·2–10 ms
2 Clinical uses (in q switched mode):
   (a) iridotomy
   (b) posterior capsulotomy
   (c) breaking of synechiae
   (d) dissection of vitreous membranes
   (e) anterior capsulotomy preoperatively
   (f) liquefaction of lens nucleus before phakoemulsification
   (g) goniotomy
   (h) breaking of vitreous strands (not if fluoride gas is in the eye)
   (i) cutting of intraocular lens loops
   (j) dispersal of preretinal haemorrhage overlying the macula in proliferative diabetic retinopathy
3 Complications:
   (a) damage to adjoining structures in the eye including endothelium, trabecular meshwork, lens, and retina
   (b) rise in intraocular pressure which may:
      (i) take several weeks to develop
      (ii) result in a pressure >50 mm Hg
      (iii) be sustained
4 Clinical uses (free running):
   (a) direct treatment to the iris causing opening up of the angle (gonioplasty) and pupil (pupilloplasty)
   (b) closing of blood vessels on iris

271

(c) trabeculoplasty
(d) trans-scleral cyclophotocoagulation
(e) irradiation of retina and choroid

Complications of laser iridotomy
1 Spontaneous closure
2 Uveitis
3 Corneal endothelial damage
4 Transient elevation of intraocular pressure
5 Permanent elevation of intraocular pressure
6 Hyphaema
7 Localised lens opacity
8 Pupillary distortion

Diode

1 Principle: 810 nm laser:
  (a) produced by semiconductor = portable and reliable
  (b) no flash = theoretically good for choroidal neovascular membrane
  (c) penetrates sclera
  (d) absorbed by blood/xanthophyll in lens
2 Uses:
  (a) cycloablation: G probe
  (b) trans-scleral diode: retinopexy probe:
    (i) retinal adhesion
    (ii) retinal ablation

Excimer lasers

1 Principle: group of lasers whose activity is related to the dissociation of a molecule of an inert gas that has been forced to associate with a molecule of a halogen gas, e.g. argon fluoride excimer laser:
  (a) emission wavelength 193 nm
  (b) photons from laser destabilise valence bonds of macromolecules causing them to fall apart
  (c) photons cannot penetrate more than a few micrometres into tissue (hence theoretically safe for use on the cornea)
  (d) excised surface is optically smooth and sealed by "pseudomembrane"
2 Uses:
  (a) fine surgical incisions in cornea (experimental)
  (b) correction of ametropia (especially myopia < –6 D) by passing laser through a circular aperture circular incisions analogous to the trephining of a lamellar bed; a 10 D negative correction can be induced by removing only 25 μm of tissue
  (c) removal of superficial corneal pathology eye, e.g. band keratopathy recurrent erosion syndrome

Complications of photorefractive keratectomy

1 Regression
2 Loss of best corrected acuity

3 Night vision problems in young patients with wide physiological mydriasis
4 Stromal scarring ("haze")
5 Anisometropia
6 Diurnal variation in visual acuity
7 Residual refractive error (i.e. over correction/under correction)

APPENDIX II

Visual standards for driving

(Adapted from the booklet *At a glance guide to the current medical standards of fitness to drive* issued by the Medical Advisory Branch of the Driver and Vehicle Licensing Agency.)

Definitions

Group 1: ordinary driving licence—private cars and motorcycles
Group 2: vocational driving licence—large goods vehicles and passenger carrying vehicles (LGV/PCV)—originally called HGV/PSV before April 1991

The table sets out the current UK regulations and national recommended guidelines for both the group 1 and 2 entitlements which are in line with the medical standards of driver licensing set out in the second EC directive. Currently a driver with a group 1 entitlement is issued with a "Till 70" years of age licence and thereafter a 3 year licence by completion of a medical questionnaire. Group 2 is usually issued to age 45 and thereafter 5 yearly until 65 when it is reviewed annually.

The law states that: a licence holder or applicant is suffering from a prescribed disability if unable to meet eyesight requirement, i.e. to read in good daylight (with the aid of spectacles or contact lenses if worn) a registration mark fixed to a motor vehicle and containing letters and figures 79·4 mm high at a distance of 20·5 m. If unable to meet this standard, the licence must be refused or revoked, and the driver must not drive.

In addition the Royal College of Ophthalmologists has issued the following guideline for the definition of the minimum field of vision necessary for safe driving:

The minimum visual field for safe driving is a field of vision of at least 120° on the horizontal measured by the Goldmann perimeter on the III4e settings (or equivalent perimetry). In addition there should be no significant field defect in the binocular field which encroaches with 20° of fixation either above or below the horizontal meridian. By this means, homonymous or bitemporal defects which come close to fixation, whether hemianopic or quadrantanopsia, are not accepted as safe for driving. Isolated scotomata represented in the binocular field near to the

VISUAL DISORDERS	GROUP 1 ENTITLEMENT	GROUP 2 ENTITLEMENT
Visual acuity Note "Grandfather" rights exist for drivers who held a Group 2 Licence prior to 1/3/92 who might be able to meet the current visual acuity standards	Must be able to meet the above requirement (in practice this corresponds to between 6/9 and 6/12 on the Snellen Chart)	New applicants are barred in law if the visual acuity using corrective lenses if necessary is worse than 6/9 in the better eye or 6/12 in the worse eye or the uncorrected visual acuity in each eye is worse than 3/60
Monocular vision Note separate regulations cover monocular drivers who held a Group 2 licence on 1/4/91 who became monocular before 1/1/91, who notified the Traffic Commissioner before this date and who have an acuity of 6/12 in the remaining eye	Need not notify DVLA if able to meet the visual acuity standard and has adapted to the disability	New applicants since 1/4/91 or existing Group 2 drivers who became monocular on or after 1/1/91 are barred in law from holding a Group 2 licence
Visual field defects For example, homonymous hemianopias and quadrantanopias, no matter which quadrant involved. Severe bilateral glaucoma, severe bilateral retinopathies (diabetes, retinitis pigmentosa). Extensive bilateral photocoagulation	Driving must cease unless confirmed able to meet the recommended national guidelines for visual fields as defined fully above	Recommended permanent refusal or revocation if associated with pathological field defects. Normal binocular vision is required for entitlement to drive these vehicles
Diplopia	Cease driving on diagnosis. May resume driving on confirmation to the DVLA that is controlled by spectacles or a patch which he undertakes to wear while driving	Recommended permanent refusal or revocation if insuperable diplopia
Night blindness For example, retinitis pigmentosa or extensive bilateral choroidoretinitis	Cease driving if unable to satisfy visual acuity and visual field requirements at all times	Driving not permitted unless able to fully meet the Group 2 eyesight requirements
Colour blindness	Need not notify DVLA. Driving may continue with no restriction on the licence	Need not notify DVLA; as for Group 1

275

Table. Approximate equivalents for common perimeters on a theoretical basis

	Perimeter	Goldmann	Cooper Dicon	Humphrey	Octopus	Fieldmaster
Target size	3/330 white	Target 4 e	—	—	—	
Angle (°)	0·52	0·7	<0·5	<0·5	<0·5	<0·5
Bowl luminance (asb)	<3	31·5	31·5	31·5	4	31·5
Target luminance (asb)	38–75	1000	315–3150	3150	Dependent on strategy and algorithm	
Target brightness over background (dB)	15	15	10–20	20	(20)	10–20

central fixation area may also be inconsistent with safe driving.

The test must therefore monitor the central area of field as well as its outer perimeter. It is obviously essential that the application of the standard should not be equipment specific and the phrase "equivalent perimetry" allows the development of equivalent programmes using other perimeters including autoperimeters (see the table below).

This definition is not statutory, but is issued by the College as advice to both the Department of Transport and the DVLA.

APPENDIX III

Definition of blindness

1 The statutory definition for the purposes of registration as a blind person under the National Assistance Act 1948 is that the person is "so blind as to be unable to perform any work for which eyesight is essential"; note:

   (a) the test is not whether the person is unable to pursue his or her ordinary occupation or any other occupation, but whether he or she is too blind to perform any work for which eyesight is essential

   (b) only the visual conditions are taken into account and other bodily or mental infirmities are disregarded

2 The principal condition to be considered is the visual acuity (i.e. the best direct vision available with each eye or both together, where both are present, as tested by Snellen's type with focus properly corrected), but regard must also be paid to the other conditions set out below

3 The persons examined may be classified in three groups as follows:

   (a) group 1: <3/60 Snellen; in general, a person with visual acuity below 3/60 may be regarded as blind

   (b) group 2: 3/60 or better, but worse than 6/60 Snellen; a person with visual acuity of 3/60 but <6/60 Snellen:

      (i) may be regarded as blind if the field of vision is considerably contracted, but

      (ii) should not be regarded as blind if the visual defect is of long standing and is unaccompanied by any material contraction of the field of vision, e.g. in cases of congenital nystagmus, albinism, myopia, etc

   (c) group 3: 6/60 Snellen or better; a person with a visual acuity of 6/60 or better should not normally be regarded as blind; he or she may, however, be regarded as blind if the field of vision is markedly contracted in the greater part of its extent, and particularly if the contraction is in the lower part of the field; however, a person suffering from homonymous or bitemporal hemianopia retaining central visual acuity of 6/18 or better is not to be regarded as blind

Notes

1 The question of whether a defect of vision is recent or of long standing has a special bearing on the certification of blindness; a person whose defect is recent is less able to adapt himself to his environment than is a person with the same visual acuity whose defect has been of long

standing; this is specially applicable to Groups 2 and 3

2 Another factor of importance, particularly in relation to Group 2, is the age of the person at the onset of blindness; an old person with a recent failure of sight cannot adapt himself so readily as can a younger person with the same defect

3 On rare occasions cases will arise which are not precisely covered by the foregoing observations, and such cases must be dealt with according to the judgment of the certifying ophthalmic surgeon

4 In making recommendations about persons up to and including the age of 16, examining ophthalmologists should bear in mind that there are other factors which may influence local education authorities in their decision about the special educational treatment to be provided

Definition of partial sight

1 There is no statutory definition in the National Assistance Act 1948 for partial sight, but the Ministry of Health has advised that the person who is not blind within the meaning of the Act 1948, but who is nevertheless substantially and permanently handicapped by congenitally defective vision, or in whose case illness or injury has caused defective vision of a substantial or permanently handicapping character is within the scope of the welfare services which the local authority are empowered to provide for blind persons; but this does not apply to other benefits specially enjoyed by the blind, e.g. Income Tax concession where eligible

2 The following criteria should be used as a general guide when determining whether a person falls within the scope of the welfare provisions for the partially sighted, as well as in recommending, where the person is under the age of 16 years of age, the appropriate type of school for the particular child concerned:

  (a) for registration purposes and the provision of welfare services, those with visual acuity:

    (i) 3/60 to 6/60 with full field

    (ii) up to 6/24 with moderate contraction of the field, opacities in media, or aphakia

    (iii) 6/18 or even better if there is a gross field defect, e.g. hemianopia, or there is a marked contraction of the field as in pigmentary degeneration, glaucoma, etc

  (b) for children whose visual acuity will have a bearing on the appropriate methods of education:

    (i) severe visual disabilities—to be educated in Special Schools by methods involving vision—3/60 to 6/24 with spectacles

    (ii) visual impairment—to be educated at ordinary schools by special consideration—better than 6/24 with spectacles

Notes

1 Infants and young children with congenital anomalies, including visual defects, unless obviously blind should be classed as being partially sighted

2 At age 4 and over, binocular corrected vision should be the criterion

3 All in (ii) of (a) and (b) above should be re-examined every 12 months, or earlier if there is reason to suspect any worsening

4 In making recommendations about persons up to and including the age of 16, examining ophthalmologists should bear in mind that—as with blindness—there are other factors which may influence local education authorities in their decision about the special education treatment to be provided

FURTHER READING

Clinical ophthalmology

Chignell AH. *Retinal detachment surgery.* 2nd edn. Berlin: Springer, 1988.

Duane TD. *Clinical ophthalmology.* Philadelphia: Harper & Row, 1986.

Spalton DJ, Hitchings RA, Hunter PA. *Atlas of clinical ophthalmology,* 2nd edn. Chicago: Mosby-Yearbook, 1993.

Kanski JJ. *Clinical ophthalmology,* 3rd edn. Oxford: Butterworth-Heinemann, 1994.

Kanski JJ, Gregor Z. *Retinal detachment: a colour manual of diagnosis and treatment,* 2nd edn. Oxford: Butterworth-Heinemann, 1995.

Kirkness CM, Seal D. *Manual of ocular infection.* Edinburgh: Churchill, 1995.

Mein J, Trimble R. *Diagnosis and management of ocular motility disorders,* 2nd edn. Oxford: Blackwell Scientific, 1991.

Newell FW. *Ophthalmology – principles and concepts,* 7th edn. Chicago: Mosby, 1992.

Taylor R, Shah P, Murray PI, Fielder A. *Key topics in ophthalmology.* Oxford: Bios Scientific, 1995.

Optics and refraction

Abrams D (ed). *Duke-Elder's practice of refraction,* 10th edn. Edinburgh: Churchill, 1993.

Elkington AR, Frank HJ. *Clinical optics,* 2nd edn. Oxford: Blackwell Scientific, 1991.

Neurology and general medicine

Ashworth B, Isherwood I. *Clinical neuro-ophthalmology.* 2nd edn. Oxford: Blackwell Scientific: 1981.

Kanski JJ, Thomas DJ. *The eye in systemic disease,* 2nd edn. Guildford: Butterworths, 1990.

Patten J. *Neurological differential diagnosis.* London: Harold Starke, 1977.

Rubinstein D, Wayne D. *Lecture notes in clinical medicine,* 4th edn. Oxford: Blackwell Scientific, 1991.

Basic sciences and pathology

Bron AJ, Marshall J, Warwick R, Tripathi R (eds) *Wolff's anatomy of the eye and orbit,* 8th edn. London: Chapman & Hall, in preparation.

Davson H. *Physiology of the eye*, 5th edn. Chicago: Macmillan, 1990.

Hart W M (ed). *Adler's physiology of the eye*, 9th edn. Chicago: Mosby/Yearbook, 1992.

Lucas DR. *Greer's ocular pathology*, 4th edn. Oxford: Blackwell Scientific, 1989.

Index